How to Survive a Catastrophic Illness Without Going Broke

SPECIAL REPORT N087

Author: Ellen Klein
Editor: Kathy A. Shipp
Editorial Director: Annette Licitra
Publisher: Philip W. Clark

Reprinted 2001.

ISBN 1-880024-48-9

Contents

Preface

'Financially, we're better off today than before John's stroke.'

In 1996 my husband suffered a massive stroke while at work. John was only 48 years old. I was 41. Neither of us had ever dealt with a medical crisis, although we'd been through the ordeal of deaths in the family. As I came to discover, a sudden medical crisis is far more difficult to handle, particularly when you're alone.

John spent about two months recovering in three hospitals and another two months in outpatient therapy five days a week, six hours a day. Because he had suffered bouts of bronchitis in previous years, he had no sick leave left, so his employer was forced to place him on leave without pay.

The stroke left John slightly paralyzed on his right side. He has difficulty walking, talking, reading, writing . . . and remembering what he did an hour ago. He did try to return to work seven months after his stroke, but it took him 24 hours to recover from each six-hour day in the office. After six weeks of trying, he conceded defeat and returned to leave-without-pay status.

Discover the Power of Cash Flow

Throughout the past 18 months, I've managed to keep my freelance writing business afloat. But as John's "primary caregiver," I now can work only about 20 hours per week instead of 60. As a result, our six-figure income has shrunk to five. Our expenses have increased some 25 percent, partly from medical bills but also because we've had to buy extras, such as educational software to help John regain his computer skills and clothing that's easier for him to put on one-handed. Yet, paradoxically, *we're financially better off today than before John's stroke.*

Not everyone we've met through John's rehabilitation program has been so fortunate. In fact, many—if not most—have lost their jobs, their homes, their life's savings—even their marriages. With insurance rules and regulations constantly changing, I can't say we won't eventually be in a similar predicament. But we do have one important advantage—**the power of cash flow**.

In this Special Report I'll share with you everything I've learned about surviving a medical crisis without going broke. It's the kind of book I wish I'd had to help me through the past year and a half. You'll learn firsthand how to mitigate financial difficulties *before* they happen—and how to tap into financial resources after a medical catastrophe occurs. Although there is no absolute safety net, this Special Report will improve your chances of landing on your feet.

What this book does not address in detail are medical catastrophes arising out of workplace incidents, automobile accidents or situations such as medical malpractice. In those cases, get yourself an attorney. Many lawyers will work on a contingent fee basis; they get paid only if you get a monetary award or settlement. But you should recognize that lawsuits take many months, even years, to pursue, and this Special Report can help you stay afloat while your claim is in litigation.

—ELLEN KLEIN

Introduction: It Could Happen to You

After years of fearing that my husband's smoking, drinking and eating habits were turning him into a stroke-waiting-to-happen, I finally decided it was more likely he'd be killed in a car accident. I was wrong. The next day, he suffered a stroke.

What Are Your Odds?

For the average American, the odds of dying this year are about 1 in 119. In contrast, the chance that you'll be hospitalized within the next 365 days is about 1 in 6. And the probability that you will be disabled for 30 or more days in the next 15 years is greater than 50 percent.

The fact is, the death rate from disease and accidents has been declining during our lifetime. Yet, ironically, due to medical and technological advances such as bypass surgery and automobile air bags, the possibility of suffering a long-term, disabling injury or illness is increasing. During the past 25 years, the number of severely disabled individuals between the ages of 17 and 44 has skyrocketed 400 percent.

Nowadays, a woman like me, age 42, has a 66 percent greater chance of surviving hypertension, heart disease, cerebrovascular disease and diabetes than my grandparents did. Although two of my grandparents never reached age 65, the chances that I'll die before age 65 are only about 14 percent; the risk that I'll be disabled 30 days or more before age 65 is greater than 40 percent.

If, like most people, you think that a disabling illness or injury is remote, consider the following statistics:

	Chances of Death Before Age 65		Chances of Disability for 30 Days or More Before Age 65	
Age	**Male**	**Female**	**Male**	**Female**
30	23.5%	16.2%	33.1%	56.6%
35	22.8	15.6	31.3	51.7
40	21.8	14.8	29.1	45.2
45	20.4	13.6	26.3	37.5
50	18.3	11.8	22.6	29.3
55	14.9	9.2	17.6	21.0
60	9.3	5.5	10.6	11.9

Source: Guardian Life Insurance Company of America

IS YOUR LIFESTYLE KILLING YOU?

At the time my husband had his stroke, I didn't know we were facing a catastrophe. After he'd been taken by ambulance to the nearest hospital and spent five hours in the emergency room, he initially was going to be sent home. On second thought, the ER doctor decided to admit John to the hospital for observation. Six hours later, he was moved to intensive care because he was having seizures. Eight days later, when the seizures had passed, an MRI revealed that he had suffered a stroke.

As I've since learned, a stroke strikes every minute in the United States, and currently 3 million Americans are permanently disabled because of stroke. Each year, 550,000 Americans experience a new or recurrent stroke. In fact, stroke is the No. 1 cause of adult disability and the third leading cause of death, affecting four out of five American families during their lifetime.

If the statistics about strokes surprise you, hold onto your socks. Every 15 seconds, someone in the United States experiences a brain injury. Motor vehicles, including motorcycles, account for nearly 50 percent of all brain injuries; falls, more than 20 percent; assault, about 10 percent; sports/recreation, 10 percent; and blunt machinery, 10 percent.

Of the more than 2 million Americans who will sustain a brain injury this year, 500,000 will have moderate to severe injuries requiring medical assistance; 373,000 will require hospitalization; 99,000 will become permanently disabled; and 2,400 will die or exist in a vegetative state. Two-thirds of them are under the age of 34: 70 percent of those are between the ages of 15 and 28 (66 percent males, 34 percent females), and the most frequent ages are 16 and 17, the time when most people get their driver's license.

OUT OF THE BLUE, INTO THE RED?

If you become disabled, how will you and your family live until you go back to work? Nearly one in five people will become disabled for five years or more during their working years, according to insurance experts. A survivor of a severe brain injury, for example, typically faces 5 to 10 years of intensive rehabilitation.

How Long Will Your Disability Last?

Age	Average Duration of Long-Term Disability*
Under age 40	4 years
40–44	4 years, 4 months
45–49	4 years, 7 months
50–54	4 years, 6 months
55–59	3 years, 6 months
60–64	1 year, 9 months

*Lasting a minimum of 90 days.

Source: Society of Actuaries Report, *Transactions* (1981)

What if you are never able to go back to work? That possibility is a lot greater than you may realize. As the chart on page 5 shows, about one in four workers ages 35 to 44 will not return to work after becoming disabled. What if that person were you? Or your spouse? Or your college-age child?

Most people will suffer serious financial hardship if their paychecks stop. If you have trouble living on two incomes now, imagine trying to live on one. A 1996 survey cited by UNUM Life Insurance Company of America revealed that the average employee has less than five weeks' worth of savings readily available. Even if you've been saving 5 percent of your income each year, a six-month disability could wipe out 10 years' worth of savings.

An illness or injury that lasts a lifetime has an even higher financial toll. Yet most people below age 65 are totally unprepared for the possibility of losing their ability to earn income. In fact, about 75 percent of employers don't offer their employees long-term disability insurance, according to the Bureau of Labor Statistics. And workers' compensation doesn't cover the majority of accidents because almost two-thirds occur off the job.

Disabled Employees Who Do Not Return to Work

Age Range	Percentage
16–34	21%
35–44	25
45–54	48
55–64	60

Source: HIAA Sourcebook of Health Insurance Data, 1996

As for throwing yourself upon the kindness of friends, can you name three people who would pay your bills for the rest of your life, without any hope of repayment?

Don't Panic

That's why we've prepared this Special Report. In Part I you'll learn why it's important to know what your health insurance covers; how much of a safety net you need; and how to compile an "Answers" file to protect your financial assets. Part II covers the process of maintaining cash flow while you're disabled; the types of help you can get when returning to work; and what to expect if you can't go back to work or will need nursing home care.

Unfortunately, about one-third of American families with an ailing family member go broke as a result of the illness. This Special Report, based on my experience, will show how you may avoid financial ruin, even when your safety net isn't entirely in place.

Part I

Prepare for the Worst, Hope for the Best

The No. 1 way to avoid financial ruin in a medical crisis is by making sure you have adequate insurance. If you have health insurance, do you know what it *doesn't* cover? You may be surprised to learn that so-called comprehensive medical policies rarely pay for health care expenses once you leave the hospital. And if you think long-term-care policies are just for senior citizens, you should know that premiums are significantly lower if you buy before age 60.

Besides insurance advice, Part I offers guidance about the tedious, yet important task of making sure your financial affairs would be handled properly if you became incapacitated. Some of this preparation involves legal paperwork, such as a durable power of attorney, but mainly it requires that you sit down and make lists that will essentially inventory your entire life.

Frankly, the amount of paperwork involved in preparing your safety net is too much to tackle all at once. So you'll want to read and reread Part I over a period of weeks as you put together your emergency plan—and even review it again in a year or so to make sure your safety net hasn't sprung leaks.

Health Insurance: What You Don't Know Can Hurt You 1

My husband's medical bills for four months' hospitalization and outpatient rehabilitation totaled more than $175,000, most of which was paid by the health insurance John had through his employer. The story could have been a lot different, though. The hospital where John was taken by ambulance didn't have a health care provider contract with his HMO. So if the emergency room physician had sent John home as originally planned, we would have been stuck with the bills for the ambulance and ER, which came to about $1,000.

John hadn't selected a primary care physician, so the HMO had to find a doctor willing to risk his "outcomes rating" by agreeing to take a critically ill patient sight-unseen. And if the HMO case manager assigned to oversee John's treatment hadn't been such a good advocate, he wouldn't have received full-time rehab—the HMO administrators kept pressuring her to cut costs by scheduling therapists to come to our home.

Can You Spare Your Life Savings?

A hospital stay typically lasts about a week and costs roughly $15,000. If you have a serious accident or illness, however, you may require hospitalization for at least seven weeks, which may run about $100,000. In fact, it's not unusual for a victim of a serious car accident to be hospitalized for six months or longer, at a cost of $350,000.

After hospitalization, you might need additional care provided in your home. The cost of visits by a registered nurse or therapist varies from state to state but can run as much as $80 for a three- or four-hour visit. Custodial caregivers and home health aides provide "nonskilled" nursing services and therefore are somewhat less expensive than RNs; they range from $40 to $60 for a three- to four-hour visit. Thus, depending on where you live and the types of services provided, a year of home health care could cost you more than $50,000. (Round-the-clock assistance could cost well over $100,000.)

Or, you might need residential or institutional care: that is, care provided in a skilled nursing facility (primarily medical/rehabilitation treatment) or a nursing home (chiefly custodial care, such as assistance with bathing, dressing and eating). Again, the costs vary widely from state to state, ranging from about $30,000 to more than $100,000 a year. Researchers in 1990 found that one out of two couples are impoverished within a year after a spouse enters a nursing home; for unmarried individuals, the rate is 7 out of 10.

Indeed, illness is said to be one of the leading causes of bankruptcy in the United States. Even if you have health care insurance (more than 40 million Americans don't), your financial security is not guaranteed: Aside from annual deductibles of up to $7,500 and/or copayments of up to 20 percent, the majority of health insurance plans have lifetime limits on benefits. Currently, between 1,500 and 2,000 people lose their private health insurance coverage each year because their expenses have exceeded $1 million (their lifetime cap). The average lifetime cost, for example, for a person who has suffered a spinal cord injury and is on a ventilator is more than $5 million.

Observation: *As of this writing, Congress is considering legislation to raise lifetime limits on health insurance benefits to $10 million by 2002. However, if health care costs continue to increase at rates far exceeding that of inflation (15.7 percent for outpatient care and 7.8 percent for inpatient care), it won't take long for even a $10 million cap to be too low.*

UNINSURED AND LIVING DANGEROUSLY

Nearly 18 percent of the U.S. population doesn't have health care coverage—not even Medicaid. The highest incidence is in the South (more than 20 percent aren't covered), and the largest category of uninsured people are ages 15 to 44 (again, more than 20 percent).

Who Isn't Covered by Health Insurance?

About 1 in 20 have incomes of at least $50,000.

About 1 in 10 have incomes of $35,000–$49,999.

Nearly 1 in 5 have incomes of $25,000–$34,999.

More than 1 in 4 have incomes of $14,000–$24,999.

More than 1 in 3 have incomes of less than $14,000.

Source: 1996 Medical Expenditure Panel Survey

The only reason to have health insurance is to protect your financial resources from being depleted in a medical emergency. If you have the money to pay for your health care, you may have decided to forgo the added expense of health insurance premiums. So-called self-insurance could make sense if you're absolutely healthy and wear a football helmet at all times. In that case, your insurance premiums *plus* lost interest or dividend income resulting from paying the premiums *plus* your insurance deductible *plus* your copayments just might exceed your actual health care costs, as in the example below:

Without insurance:	
National average annual health care expenses per person	**$3,510**
With insurance:	
National average individual health care policy	$2,500
+ 6 percent return on $2,500 if it were invested (.06 × 2,500)	150
+ annual insurance deductible	500
+ 20 percent copayment for expenses over $500 (.20 × 3,010)	602
Average annual health care expenses per person	**$3,752**
Self-insurance savings per year	**$242**

Over a 20-year period, assuming you spend the annual average on health care and never remove your football helmet, you'd save about $5,000. If you never go to a doctor at all, and therefore save $3,510 per year, you would amass more than $70,000 (not including interest) in savings by the end of 20 years. Of course, one serious accident or illness could wipe out all that you've saved—as well as the rest of your assets. Is this a risk you really want to take?

NOT EVERYONE QUALIFIES FOR MEDICAID

Lots of people think it's OK not to have health insurance because they assume that Medicaid is a guaranteed safety net. It's not.

"Medicaid does *not* provide medical assistance for all poor persons," warned Mary Onnis Waid of the federal Health Care Financing Administration. "Even under the broadest provisions of the federal statute, Medicaid does not provide health care services even for the very poor *unless* they are in one of the groups designed [by law]."

States generally have broad discretion in determining which groups their Medicaid programs will cover and the financial criteria for Medicaid eligibility, Waid said. However, to be eligible for federal Medicaid funds, states are required to provide at least some Medicaid coverage for certain **"categorically needy"** eligibility groups. These include:

- ✔ All recipients of Temporary Assistance to Needy Families (TANF). TANF replaced the open-ended federal entitlement program known as Aid to Families with Dependent Children (AFDC). TANF limits a family's lifetime cash welfare benefits to five years.
- ✔ Families who lose TANF because of money from child support collections or increased earnings. They are automatically eligible for several months after losing TANF benefits.
- ✔ Pregnant women (single or married) whose income is at or below 133 percent of the Federal Poverty Income Guidelines *(see box at right)*. Once eligible for Medicaid, they remain eligible throughout the pregnancy and up to 60 days thereafter. Services covered may be limited to pregnancy, complications of pregnancy, delivery and postpartum care.
- ✔ Supplemental Security Income (SSI) recipients in most states. (Some states use more restrictive Medicaid eligibility requirements that predate SSI.)

Federal Poverty Income Guidelines*

Family Size	Annual	Monthly	133% (Monthly)	170% (Monthly)
1	$ 7,890	$ 658	$ 874	$1,118
2	10,610	884	1,176	1,503
3	13,330	1,111	1,477	1,888
4	16,050	1,338	1,779	2,274
5	18,770	1,564	2,080	2,659
6	21,490	1,791	2,382	3,044
7	24,210	2,018	2,683	3,430
8	26,930	2,244	2,985	3,815
Additional Person	2,720	227	301	385

*Effective through March 31, 1998

✔ Certain beneficiaries of Medicare.

✔ Children under age 21 who are in foster care or subsidized adoptions.

✔ Certain people who lost SSI because their income or living situation changed.

✔ Infants born to Medicaid-eligible women. The infants are covered until their first birthday if their mothers remain eligible.

✔ Children younger than age 6 whose family income is at or below 133 percent of the Federal Poverty Income Guidelines.

✔ Children ages 6 to 19 whose family income is at or below 100 percent of the Federal Poverty Income Guidelines.

About the 'Medically Needy' Program

Under the Medically Needy (MN) program states have the option of extending Medicaid eligibility to additional qualified persons. These persons would be eligible for Medicaid under one of the mandatory or optional groups, except that their income/resources are above the eligibility level set by their state. MN income levels (for example, $2,000 for an individual; $3,000 for a couple) are higher than the regular Medicaid eligibility income levels.

If a state elects to have any MN program, it must include certain groups and services: children under age 19 and pregnant women who are medically needy, as well as prenatal and delivery care and ambulatory care for children.

Persons may immediately qualify or may "spend down" by incurring medical expenses that place them at or below their state's MN income level. For medically needy adults, resources that *do not count* against the income limit include:

- Your house and the lot, plus $5,000 worth of land around the house and the lot.
- Up to $2,500 set aside for burial expenses if you are elderly, blind or disabled.
- One automobile.

Resources that *do count* against the income limit include:

- Money on hand, in the bank or in a safe deposit box.
- Stocks, bonds and certificates of deposit.
- Refundable prepaid burial accounts and plans (unless designated as an allowable burial set-aside).
- The value of more than one motor vehicle.
- The cash value of life insurance (on a person age 21 or older) with a face value of more than $1,500.
- The amount still owed on a deed of trust or mortgage when you hold the note and are due the payments.
- Any property that is inherited.

Observation: *A 1987 study by the U.S. House Select Committee on Aging found that after only 13 weeks (91 days), 7 in 10 elderly people living alone spent down their income to federal poverty levels.*

In addition, states have the *option* of providing Medicaid coverage for other **"categorically related"** groups. These optional groups share the characteristics of the mandatory groups, but the eligibility criteria are somewhat more liberal. The broadest optional groups for which states will receive federal matching funds for coverage under the Medicaid program include:

✔ Infants up to age 1 and pregnant women not covered under the mandatory rules whose family income is no more than 185 percent of the Federal Poverty Income Guidelines (the percentage is set by each state).

✔ Children under age 21 who meet what were the AFDC income and resources requirements in effect in their state on July 16, 1996 (even though they do not meet the mandatory eligibility requirements).

✔ Individuals who would be eligible if institutionalized, but who are receiving care under home and community-based services waivers.

✔ Institutionalized individuals eligible under a special income level (the amount is set by each state—up to 300 percent of the SSI federal benefits rate).

✔ Recipients of state supplementary income payments.

✔ TB-infected persons who would be financially eligible for Medicaid at the SSI income level if they were within a Medicaid-covered category. However, eligibility is only for TB-related ambulatory services and for TB drugs.

✔ Certain elderly, blind or disabled adults who have incomes above those requiring mandatory coverage but below the Federal Poverty Income Guidelines.

✔ "Medically needy" persons. *(See box on page 12.)*

If your state determines that you are eligible for Medicaid, coverage generally is retroactive to the third month prior to your application. Your coverage generally stops at the end of the month in which you no longer meet the criteria of any Medicaid eligibility group.

MEDICAID WON'T COVER EVERYTHING

Medicaid does not necessarily cover all the kinds of medical treatment you might require. State Medicaid programs must offer medical assistance for only certain basic services. These services generally include:

- Inpatient hospital services.
- Prenatal care.
- Physician services.
- Family planning services and supplies.
- Home health care for persons eligible for skilled nursing services.
- Outpatient hospital services.
- Vaccines for children.
- Nursing facility services for persons age 21 or older.
- Rural health clinic services.
- Laboratory and X-ray services.
- Nurse-midwife services.

- Federally qualified health center (FQHC) services and ambulatory services of an FQHC that would be available in other settings.
- Early and periodic screening, diagnostic and treatment (EPSDT) services for children under age 21.
- Pediatric and nurse practitioner services.

States may also receive federal matching funds for providing certain optional services, most commonly the following:

- Diagnostic services.
- Intermediate care facilities for the mentally retarded.
- Optometrist services and eyeglasses.
- Home and community-based care for some with chronic impairments.
- Clinic services.
- Prescribed drugs and prosthetic devices.
- Transportation services.
- Nursing facility services for children under age 21.
- Rehabilitation and physical therapy.

Within broad federal guidelines, states determine the amount and duration of services offered under their Medicaid programs. They may limit, for example, the number of days of hospital care or the number of doctor visits covered. Also, Medicaid does not cover services received from providers who are not enrolled in the state's Medicaid program or who will not accept Medicaid rates as payment in full.

Caution: *Don't assume that your local hospital participates in your state's Medicaid program—or, if it does, that it is approved to provide the services you need.* Prior to the spring of 1986, for example, Mount Vernon Hospital in Fairfax County, Virginia, which offers one of the best inpatient rehabilitation programs in the nation, was approved only as an acute-care hospital. This meant it was subject to the state's Medicaid regulation limiting payment for hospitalization to 21 days. The nearest Medicaid-approved long-term-care facility was in Richmond, about two hours away by car. It took extensive lobbying on behalf of a teenager who had suffered a traumatic brain injury in a car accident—and ultimately an emergency resolution by the governor of Virginia—for the hospital to be approved as a Medicaid provider of inpatient rehabilitation.

MEDICAID CAN HAVE (PURSE)STRINGS ATTACHED

States are permitted to require some Medicaid recipients to pay deductibles, co-insurance or copayments for certain services. In addition, you will be expected to pay for any services you receive that are not covered by Medicaid (such as a heart transplant if you are older than 21) or that exceed the Medicaid limit for that service (for example, hospitalization beyond a 21-day period). Routine copay amounts are $1 per office visit or $3 per other visit; $1 per prescription; and $100 per inpatient hospitalization.

Many people don't consider applying for Medicaid until they face the need for long-term nursing home care, of which Medicaid pays about 42 percent of the cost. However, even after you become eligible for Medicaid, most of your income must be used to pay toward the cost of care in the nursing facility. This is called your "patient pay," which Medicaid supplements up to the cost of care.

In 1988 Congress passed provisions to prevent what has come to be called "spousal impoverishment," leaving the spouse who is still living at home with little or no income or resources. The provisions apply when one's spouse is expected to remain in a nursing facility or medical institution for at least 30 days. When the couple applies for Medicaid, an assessment of their resources is made. The couple's resources are combined, with exemptions given for the home, household goods, an automobile and burial funds. The result is the spousal resource amount, which is the minimum resource standard ($16,152 in 1998); or the spousal share, which is equal to one-half of the couple's combined resources, not to exceed the maximum permitted by federal law ($80,760 in 1998). Although the resource allowance goes up every year, pegged to inflation, keep in mind that states can set their own limits within this range. All resources held by both spouses are considered as being available to the spouse in the medical facility, except for the share attributed to the spouse who is still living at home.

What if there are assets above the limits? To a certain extent, the assets may be legally transferred or protected within a Medicaid-qualifying trust. For example, you might convert liquid savings into equity in a house by paying down the mortgage, adding improvements to an existing home or even buying a larger house.

Be careful with asset transfers

Caution: *Do not attempt to transfer or shield assets without substantial review with a competent adviser.* States are required to withhold payment for various long-term-care services if you dispose of assets for less than fair market value. States can "look back" to find such asset transfers for 36 months prior to the date you are institutionalized or, if later, the date you apply for Medicaid. For certain trusts, the "look-back" period extends to 60 months.

In addition, under federal law, anyone who tries to get the government to pay for his health care when, in fact, he is not eligible for government benefits is committing fraud and possibly embezzlement, which is a felony punishable by fine as well as imprisonment. These penalties also apply to any professional (including a lawyer or a financial adviser) who advises you about ways to transfer your assets to become eligible for Medicaid.

If a state uncovers a transfer of assets for less than fair market value, it must withhold payment for certain long-term-care services for a "penalty period." The length of the penalty period is determined by dividing the value of the transferred asset by the average monthly private-pay rate for nursing facility care in the state. For example, a transferred asset worth $90,000, divided by a $3,000 average monthly private-pay rate, results in a 30-month penalty period. There is no limit to the length of the penalty period.

Penalties do not apply to certain types of transfers, principally:

- Transfers to a spouse or to a third party for the sole benefit of the spouse.
- Transfers by a spouse to a third party for the sole benefit of the spouse.
- Transfers to certain disabled individuals or to trusts established for those individuals.
- Transfers for a purpose other than to qualify for Medicaid.
- Transfers where imposing a penalty would cause undue hardship.

Another issue to consider is that you might have to pay considerable gift taxes on the transfer: anything over $10,000 that you transfer to an individual per year or over your lifetime gift tax exemption of $625,000 is subject to gift tax. (Note that the $625,000 lifetime exemption in effect in 1998 is scheduled to increase gradually to $1 million by 2006.)

How a trust is treated depends to some extent on what type of trust it is (revocable or irrevocable) and what specific requirements and conditions the trust contains. In general, however, payments actually made to you or for your benefit are treated as income.

Amounts that could be paid to you or for your benefit—but are not—are treated as available resources. Amounts that could be paid to you or for your benefit but are paid to someone else are treated as transfers of assets for less than fair market value. Amounts that cannot, in any way, be paid to you or for your benefit are also treated as transfers of assets for less than fair market value.

Estate Recovery Provision

The Omnibus Budget Reconciliation Act of 1993 requires each state to seek adjustment or recovery of amounts paid by the state for certain Medicaid beneficiaries. At a minimum, the state must seek recovery for services provided to a person of any age in a nursing facility, intermediate care facility for the mentally retarded or other medical institution. The state may also, at its option, recover amounts up to the total amount spent on the individual's behalf for medical assistance for other services.

For individuals age 55 or older, states are required to seek recovery of payments from the individual's estate for nursing facility services, home and community-based services, and related hospital and prescription drug services. States also have the option of recovering payments for all other Medicaid services provided to these individuals.

In addition, states that had Medicaid plans approved after May 14, 1993, which disregarded assets or resources of persons with long-term-care insurance policies, must recover all Medicaid costs for nursing facility and other long-term-care services from those persons' estates. California, Connecticut, Indiana, Iowa and New York are exempt from this requirement because they had state plans approved prior to May 14, 1993.

The types of trusts that don't affect your Medicaid eligibility include:

- ❑ Trusts established by a parent, grandparent, guardian or court for an individual who is disabled and under the age of 65, using the individual's own funds.
- ❑ Trusts established by a disabled individual, parent, grandparent, guardian or court for a disabled individual, using the individual's own funds, where the trust is made up of pooled funds and managed by a nonprofit organization for the sole benefit of each individual included in the trust.
- ❑ Trusts composed only of pension, Social Security and other income of the individual, in states that make individuals eligible for institutional care under a special income level but do not cover institutional care for the medically needy.

Caution: *In all the instances where trusts are not counted as being available to the individual, the trust must provide that the state will receive any funds (up to the amount of Medicaid benefits paid on behalf of the individual) remaining in the trust when the individual dies.*

GOING THE PRIVATE INSURANCE ROUTE

Aside from eligibility issues, co-insurance amounts and availability of Medicaid-approved health care facilities, another drawback to relying on Medicaid is that too often "you get what you pay for." Recent government surveys reveal that, among Medicaid beneficiaries, there's significant dissatisfaction with the level of service and quality of care provided. If this gives you pause—and it should, if for no other reason than the fact that poor treatment of your illness or injury could prolong your inability to work—you should consider going the private insurance route. Generally speaking, there are two ways to obtain private health care insurance: through a group or on your own.

Group health insurance is typically offered through employers, unions, professional associations and other organizations. Frequently, the premiums are lower than those of individual insurance because economies of scale in large groups make administration less expensive.

With group insurance, if you enroll when you first become eligible for coverage, you generally will not be asked for proof that you are insurable. Enrollment usually occurs when you first take a job or during a specified period each year, which is called "open enrollment."

Individual health insurance allows you to choose your insurance company and select a plan that best fits your needs. It requires careful shopping, however, because coverage and costs vary from company to company.

Note: If you find it difficult to get insurance on your own, check with your state insurance department to see if your state has a risk pool. Similar to risk pools for automobile insurance, these can provide insurance for people who cannot get it elsewhere.

Health plans fall into two broad categories: fee-for-service (indemnity) and managed care plans.

Fee-for-service plans let you choose your doctors, hospitals and other health care providers. You or the provider sends the bill to the insurance company, which pays a portion of it. Usually you have an annual deductible, such as $200, before the insurer starts paying. Once you satisfy the deductible, the insurer typically pays 80 percent of what it considers the "usual and customary" charge for covered services, while you pay the other 20 percent, called your "co-insurance" amount. However, if the provider charges

How the Health Insurance Law Affects You

Popularly known as the Kennedy/Kassebaum Bill, the Health Insurance Portability and Accountability Act of 1996 is intended to ensure access to health insurance for people who have had coverage but want to change jobs or start a business of their own. **But beware:** *All you get under the new law is access to coverage. There's no guarantee that the coverage will be affordable.*

As of July 1, 1997, insurers may impose only one 12-month waiting period for any pre-existing condition treated or diagnosed in the previous six months. Your prior insurance coverage will be credited toward that waiting period, provided you have maintained continuous coverage without a break of more than 62 days. If you change jobs, your new employer can limit you to the type of coverage you had previously—even if other employees are receiving additional coverage. For example, if your old plan didn't cover prescription drugs, your new plan isn't required to offer it to you.

What if your new company has no health plan or you go into business for yourself? The law requires that you have unrestricted access to a choice of individual policies if you previously had insurance for at least 18 months and you are coming out of a group health plan.

more than what the insurer considers the "usual and customary" charge, you will have to pay both the co-insurance and the difference.

Managed care plans come in three basic flavors: Preferred Provider Organization (PPO), Health Maintenance Organization (HMO) and Point-of-Service (POS) plans:

- **A PPO has arrangements with doctors, hospitals and other health care providers** who agree to accept lower fees from the insurer for their services. If you go to a doctor within the PPO network, you will pay a set amount for certain services (copayment), such as $10 for a doctor visit or $5 for a prescription, and a lower co-insurance. If you go to a health care provider outside the network, you will have to meet the deductible and pay co-insurance based on higher charges. In addition, you may have to pay the difference between what the provider charges and what the plan will pay.
- **HMOs offer a range of health benefits for a set monthly fee.** If doctors are employees of the health plan and you visit them at central medical facilities or clinics, it is known as a staff or group model HMO. Other HMOs contract with physician groups or individual doctors who have private offices—these are called individual practice associations (IPAs) or networks. In either case, the HMO will give you a list of doctors from which to choose a primary care physician. This doctor is considered the "gatekeeper," meaning that you'll usually have to contact her to be referred to a specialist.

  With some HMOs, you pay nothing when you use the health care services. Other HMOs require a copayment of $5 or $10 for some services. Of course, the plan covers only the charges for providers in that plan; if you go outside the plan, you will have to pay the bill.
- **Many HMOs offer an option known as a POS plan,** in which you can refer yourself to a provider outside the plan and still get some coverage; that is, you will have to pay co-insurance. But if the primary care doctor in the POS plan makes a referral outside the network, the plan will pay most or all of the bill.

What you need to know about managed care

Managed care plans (most frequently referred to as HMOs) have been able to slow down the rapid increase in health care costs by instituting a system that essentially rewards doctors and other health care providers who do not "overutilize" expensive services, such as inpatient hospitalization and high-tech diagnostics. Indeed, managed care came about, in large part, because of the perception that many fee-for-service providers were fattening their incomes by performing unnecessary tests and surgeries.

The way managed care plans curtail wasteful expenditures of medical resources is by paying providers a set fee, based on the number of members (patients) the provider is expected to serve. If the provider sees a patient every week or once a year, the fee is the same. Obviously, the less time and resources the provider spends on each patient, the higher that provider's net income will be.

Unfortunately, this method of payment, known as **capitation**, has had some serious side effects. Some doctors continued to behave as if they were fee-for-service providers, making extensive referrals for testing and surgeries. This led to what has been called the "gag rule," by which managed care plans sought to prevent doctors from discussing expensive treatment options with their patients. It also led to preauthorization requirements, whereby doctors' referrals first had to be approved by administrators of the managed care plan. A major consequence of these rules has been the denial of costly treatments; in other words, medical rationing.

Managed care plans have been allowed to perfect the art of medical rationing because they have been protected from malpractice suits under the federal Employee Retirement Income Security Act of 1974 (ERISA). The law was originally written to protect the integrity of pension plans, but its provisions cover all company benefits, including health insurance. Under ERISA, claims against company health plans have to be brought in federal court. But malpractice is a state offense and therefore cannot be brought in federal court.

The issue of how to hold a health care insurer liable for denying patients critical treatment has gained significant attention across the country. In May 1997 Texas passed the first state law allowing patients to bring malpractice claims against HMOs and other managed care plans. In June 1997 Missouri achieved a similar result by making it clear that HMOs practice medicine and therefore are open to malpractice claims. Federal courts have also taken up the issue, and now you can sue HMOs in Delaware, New Jersey, Pennsylvania, Colorado, Kansas, New Mexico, Oklahoma, Utah and Washington.

With specific regard to medical rationing, at least 20 states now allow women in managed care plans to see gynecologists and obstetricians without first getting another doctor's permission. In at least 17 states, HMOs now have to pay for emergency treatment at nonmember hospitals if a "prudent person" (as opposed to a medical expert) would think a real danger existed. Gag rules are now illegal in at least 20 states, and as of 1998, federal law requires coverage for hospital stays of up to 48 hours for normal births and 96 hours for Caesareans.

Questions to Ask Before Selecting Managed Care

Managed care plans tend to be the least expensive private insurance you can obtain. But there are tradeoffs. Before opting for managed care over fee-for-service, ask yourself the following:

1. How comprehensive do I want my health coverage to be? For example, will the insurance plan pay for prescription drugs and durable medical equipment (such as wheelchairs)?

2. How do I feel about limits on my choice of doctors or hospitals? This may be an important factor if your current physician is not a member of the managed care plan you are considering.

3. How do I feel about a primary care doctor referring me to specialists? If you want to see a dermatologist for a skin condition, for example, are you willing to take the extra step of getting a referral first—and willing to forgo the consultation if your primary care physician says it's not necessary?

4. How convenient does my care need to be? Are you willing to travel a longer distance to see an in-plan physician to pay lower premiums?

5. How important is the cost of services? Are you concerned that a $5 doctor visit will be less thorough than a $250 fee-for-service visit?

6. How much am I willing to spend on premiums and other health care costs? Remember, you may be able to deduct a portion or even all of your medical premiums and health care expenses on your income tax return.

7. How do I feel about keeping receipts and filing claims? If this is a problem for you, then a managed care plan is more your style.

HOW TO COMPARE HEALTH CARE PLANS

Once you've decided which type of insurance you want—fee-for-service or managed care—you should compare several plans and decide which benefits are most important to you. Among factors to consider are the services offered, choice of providers, location, costs and quality of care.

Look at the services offered by each plan. What services are limited or not covered? Is there a good match between what is provided and what you think you might need? For example, if your family has a history of diabetes, will the plan pay for nutrition counseling? (Many don't.) Blood testing supplies and equipment if you are not insulin dependent? (Most don't.) Or preventive foot care provided more frequently than every two months? (Some don't.)

Few fee-for-service and managed care plans cover treatments that are experimental. Ask how the plan decides what is "experimental" and what you can do if you disagree with the plan's decision.

How much choice would you have in terms of the doctors, hospitals and other medical providers who are part of the plan? Are there enough of the kinds of doctors you may want to see? Do you need to choose a primary care doctor? If you want to see a specialist, can you refer yourself or must your primary care physician refer you? Do you need the plan's approval before going into the hospital or getting specialty care?

Are the providers' locations near where you work or live? How does the plan handle care when you are away from home?

As for costs, are there deductibles you must pay before the insurance begins to help cover expenses? After you've met your deductible, what part of the cost is paid by the plan? Does this amount vary by the type of service, doctor or health care facility you use? Are there copayments for certain services? If you use doctors outside the plan's network,

Medical Savings Accounts

The federal government is conducting a demonstration project involving Medical Savings Accounts (MSAs) for people who have health insurance coverage with a high deductible ($1,500 to $2,250 for individuals; $3,000 to $4,500 for families). Approximately 750,000 taxpayers will be able to participate in this demonstration.

With MSAs, certain uninsured individuals, self-employed individuals and those employed by participating employers can deposit a certain sum every year to be used for medical bills. The money is tax free and accrues interest. Any money not spent on medical bills can be carried forward from year to year, with no taxes owed on the earnings in the account.

The law allows participants to spend their MSAs on anything they want. However, if the money is spent on something other than medical expenses, the withdrawal is subject to income tax and, if the participant is not 65 or older, a 15 percent penalty.

Once the threshold level of 750,000 taxpayers is reached, no more MSAs can be opened, at least until the year 2000, but existing participants will be able to continue making contributions to their accounts. During the blackout period, the government will evaluate the program to see whether MSAs enable more people to afford health insurance.

how much more will you pay to get care? If a plan excludes certain services or care that you think you might need, how much will you have to pay out of pocket? Are there limits to how much you must pay in case of major illness (catastrophic care)? Is there a limit on how much the plan will pay for your care in a year or over a lifetime?

Your state department of health or insurance commission may have information about the plans you're interested in. Also, several national organizations review and accredit plans and health care institutions and can tell you if a plan you are considering, or an institution in the plan, is accredited.

Some managed care plans and independent organizations are compiling "report cards," which often include results of surveys asking members about their health care experiences. The report card may also indicate whether the plan provides preventive care or follows up on test results; how many members stay in or leave the plan; how many of the plan's doctors are board certified; or how long you may have to wait for an appointment. You should also keep an eye out for magazine articles that rate health plans.

Time to Inspect Your Safety Net

2

My husband always considered "money management" ideally suited to my temperament. So even before his stroke, I did most of the household budgeting, retirement planning, tax filing and general fretting over our finances. As a result, when he became hospitalized, I had a pretty good idea of how much money was available, what income was due from various sources and what bills to expect in the coming months.

Aside from having accumulated a short-term "emergency fund," I was particularly glad that, two years before John's illness, I had bought disability income insurance and long-term-care policies for both of us. John's policies ended up paying out significantly more than we had paid in. Within six months of John's stroke, we had three times as much money in the bank as when he had gone into the hospital.

The Importance of Cash Flow

Do you have enough ready money to cover all the bills coming due in the next 12 months? Better yet, you should have enough assets that can be converted into cash to tide you over for 18 to 24 months. This may sound excessive—particularly if you're living from paycheck to paycheck—but it can often take a year and a half before workers' comp or Social Security disability benefits kick in. Meanwhile, your family will insist on eating, and your creditors on being paid. To avoid starving your loved ones and stiffing your creditors, you should make sure your usable assets are greater than your liabilities for the next 12 to 24 months.

Your usable assets can be divided into three categories: **(1) ready cash,** such as savings and checking accounts, and readily salable personal property; **(2) restricted-access assets,** such as certificates of deposit and retirement accounts, for which you may have early-withdrawal penalties; and **(3) slow- or hard-to-access assets,** such as real estate and valuable personal property, which could take awhile to sell. You should leave out of your calculations any property you want to keep, such as a car, your house and family heirlooms. You can use the following lists as a guide in adding up your usable assets:

Readily Available Assets

- Money in checking, savings and money market accounts
- Payments due you for work performed
- Available sick leave, vacation time and other paid leave
- Mutual funds, stocks, Savings Bonds, Treasury bills and other easily salable investments
- Jewelry, silver, cars and other easily salable personal property

Gold
Assets held in trusts

Restricted-Access Assets

Certificates of deposit, if early withdrawal would result in penalties
Retirement accounts, such as IRAs, Keoghs, company thrift accounts, from which you can borrow
Vested amount in your pension fund
Life insurance cash value
Employee or executive stock options

Slow- or Hard-to-Access Assets

Coin and stamp collections
Art and antiques
Real estate other than your home
Valuable personal property, such as boats and furs
Equity value of your business
Money owed to you on notes or loans

Caution: *You may be tempted to look to your credit cards, home equity value or personal (unsecured) lines of credit as potential sources of emergency funds.* Going this route is only risking more financial trouble since these loans will need to be paid back—with interest. Even if your disability is caused by someone else—say a collision with a drunken driver—don't count on winning huge (or even moderate) damages with which to pay back the loans. In some states there are almost as many uninsured motorists on the road as those who are insured. Moreover, you may run out of available credit long before your lawsuit is resolved. If you must borrow money, it is better to ask your relatives for a long-term loan, which can be forgiven or paid out of workers' comp, Social Security or other benefits you may eventually receive.

Next, you should calculate your liabilities. These can also be divided into three categories: **(1) your expected expenses** for the next 12 months or more; **(2) estimated fees and commissions, early withdrawal penalties and taxes** on assets you may need to liquidate; and **(3) guesstimated uninsured medical expenses**. You can use the following lists as a guide in adding up your liabilities:

Expected Expenses for the Next 12 Months

Auto insurance
Birthdays/holidays
Bus/subway/taxi
Charitable contributions
Clothing/shoes
Dental insurance
Doctor/dentist
Entertainment
Gas/electricity/water
Groceries/drinks/paper goods
Homeowner's insurance
Housecleaning
Laundry/dry cleaning
Long-term-care insurance
Auto loan/lease
Books/magazines
Cable TV/satellite TV
Child care/support
Credit card payments
Disability insurance
Elder care/support
Furniture/household furnishings
Gasoline
Health insurance
Home security system
Incidental expenses
Life insurance
Mortgage/rent

Other insurance
Other travel (not vacation related)
Repairs/upkeep
Retirement fund contributions
Sports/hobbies
Vacations
Other loans
Personal care
Restaurants
School/college
Telephone (residential and mobile)
Veterinarian/kennel

Taxes and Penalties

Early withdrawal penalties on CDs, IRAs, retirement funds
Fees/commissions
Federal/state capital gains taxes
Federal/state income taxes on tax-deferred contributions or earnings withdrawn from your pension plan to pay medical expenses

Uninsured Medical Expenses

Copayments/co-insurance
Deductibles
Difference between covered amount and actual charges
Medical treatments not covered by insurance
Other uninsured medical expenses
Prescriptions/medical equipment/supplies not covered by insurance

➤ **Recommendation:** *It's impossible to know what your potential uninsured medical expenses may be. However, there are two steps you can take to make an educated guess. First, carefully review your health care policy's covered expenses, payment limits, exclusions and stop-loss provisions (annual/lifetime caps on your out-of-pocket expenses). Second, call your local hospital, nearest nursing home and, if available, a physician referral service to find out what the "customary and usual" charges are for hospitalization, nursing care and doctor exams, consultations and office treatments.*

Your insurance agent may be another source of information about "customary and usual" charges in your local area. (In fact, this is a good reason to use an agent who lives in your community.) These exercises will also help you determine whether you need different or additional insurance, as discussed later in this section.

Although you can't predict what illness or medical disorder you might experience someday, you can take a realistic look at your risk factors. For example, your age, sex and family's medical history can have a large impact on your vulnerability to certain diseases. *(See box on page 27.)*

You're also in the best position to know whether your occupation or lifestyle is fraught with risks that may result in a serious illness or injury. For instance, if your job involves removing asbestos from buildings or flying experimental planes or repairing power lines, you're exposed to greater hazards than if you're a newspaper editor, kindergarten teacher or *cordon bleu* chef. Likewise, if you smoke cigarettes, use illegal intravenous drugs or drive without a seatbelt, your habits increase your respective risk of cancer, AIDS or traumatic brain injury.

Observation: *In preparing our own financial safety net for my husband and myself, I used several worst-case assumptions. First, I recognized that my husband had 9 out of the 12 risk factors for stroke. So I did all my calculations for John under the working assumption that he would suffer a permanently disabling stroke. This meant ensuring that we would have sufficient funds to provide for his long-term nursing care as well as to help pay our bills during his convalescence.*

With regard to myself, I theorized that I'd get hit by a bus and be left in a "persistent vegetative state" (motor vehicle accidents being the leading cause of traumatic brain injury, including coma). This, too, meant ensuring that we would have enough funds to provide for my long-term care and help make up for the loss of my income.

Now, to determine whether your financial safety net is strong and secure—or limp and leaky—use the following work sheet to see how your assets compare with your liabilities:

If You're Disabled by Illness or Accident (as of today's date):

Your Usable Assets		
Readily available assets	$________	
Restricted-access assets	$________	
Slow- or hard-to-access assets	$________	
Total usable assets		**$________**
Your Liabilities		
Expected expenses for the next 12 months	$________	
Taxes, fees/commissions and penalties	$________	
Uninsured medical expenses	$________	
Total liabilities		**$________**

If the amount of your total usable assets is less than your total liabilities, you're courting financial ruin. You should consult a financial professional to see how you can increase your assets and decrease your expenses. Even more important, you should talk to an insurance agent to see how you can fill some of the gaps in your financial safety net. In particular, unless you are retired, it is essential that you purchase **disability income insurance**.

Disability Insurance Protects Your Most Important Asset

Your ability to earn income to pay for your house, car and living expenses is your most important asset. Yet only about one in four workers has disability income insurance, which ensures continuation of your income in the event that an illness or injury makes it impossible for you to work (at least temporarily). If you are a single parent supporting a child, the need to protect your income is especially critical.

Example: A 30-year-old making $50,000 a year, working to age 65 and never getting a raise, will earn $1.75 million by retirement. With a 4 percent yearly raise, the income he would earn by age 65 would be $3.83 million. That's a lot of money *not* to protect.

Most people think about buying life insurance. But if you have an injury or illness that keeps you out of the work force, the consequences could be even worse than if you had died. With death, income stops—but so do the expenses of the deceased. With disability, income stops—while medical bills and other new expenses keep piling up.

Some employers offer **group disability insurance**. These plans, which may cover short-term and long-term disabilities, are usually less expensive than individual policies. However, if you pay the premiums out of pretax income or your employer pays the premiums for you, the benefits are taxable. This means that if your policy pays 60 percent of your salary, your after-tax benefit will be only 39 percent after taxes (assuming a 21 percent tax bracket). Most plans have a maximum monthly benefit of $5,000 or less, which could mean that you receive an even smaller percentage of your income. For higher wage earners, it's a good idea to have a supplemental policy to make sure you have enough coverage.

Group **short-term disability insurance** generally starts paying the first day for an accident and the eighth day for an illness. Such plans may pay benefits for 13 to 52 weeks, although most cover you for 26 weeks. Usually, though, these plans will not pay if you are receiving workers' compensation.

Group **long-term disability insurance** offers coverage that lasts beyond six months. If your employer offers it, you should take it. Most group long-term disability policies provide benefits for the first two years if you are unable to perform your regular job. But if you are still disabled after two years, the definition changes and benefits are paid only if you can't perform any job "for which you are suited by education, training or experience"—a much more restrictive definition.

Some group long-term disability policies, often called **catastrophic disability** or **permanent disability insurance**, will pay up to 100 percent income replacement if you suffer a severe, irreversible disability that not only prevents you from working but also limits your daily activities, such as bathing, dressing and eating.

Group long-term disability policies may offer you several optional benefits. For example, a **convertibility provision** enables you to convert your group coverage to an individual policy after termination of your employment. **Spousal coverage,** another option, recognizes the fact that a healthy employee whose spouse is severely disabled can still face financial hardship: the possible loss of a second income as well as the potential expense of long-term care and child care. Still another option may be a **monthly annuity premium benefit**. This feature pays your pension contributions in addition to your disability income benefits. Many policies also give you the option of buying more insurance. Buying extra coverage through a group plan is almost always less expensive than buying an individual policy.

Risk Factors at a Glance

Disorders That Occur More Frequently After Middle Age

Alzheimer's disease	Arteriosclerosis	Cancer
Diabetes	Glaucoma	Gout
High blood pressure	Osteoarthritis	Osteoporosis
Parkinson's disease		

Disorders That Strike Men More Frequently Than Women

- Arteriosclerosis prior to age 50
- Cancer of the esophagus, kidneys, larynx, lips, tongue, pharynx (throat), stomach

Disorders That Strike Women More Frequently Than Men

- Breast cancer
- Carpal tunnel syndrome
- Graves disease (overfunction of thyroid gland)
- Multiple sclerosis
- Myasthenia gravis (autoimmune disorder that causes weakness of muscles controlling swallowing and breathing)
- Osteoporosis
- Rheumatoid arthritis
- Systematic lupus erythematosus
- Thyroid cancer

Medical Conditions That Seem to Run in Families

Alzheimer's disease	Arteriosclerosis
Breast cancer	Colon and rectal cancer
Diabetes	Emphysema
High blood pressure	Prostate cancer

Note: Adapted from *Symptoms* by Isadore Rosenfeld (Simon and Schuster, 1989)

To determine if you need additional disability insurance, use the work sheet below:

Monthly take-home pay	$__________	
(minus)		
Job-related expenses (commuting, lunches, etc.)	$__________	*(Subtotal 1)*
Monthly group disability benefits (enter the after-tax amount)	$__________	
(plus)		
Other monthly disability insurance (if you have any)	$__________	*(Subtotal 2)*
Additional monthly benefit needed (Subtotal 1 *minus* Subtotal 2)	$__________	

Note: You don't have to figure taxes on this additional benefit because benefits you pay for yourself are tax free.

Generally, you will be able to choose a waiting (elimination) period, ranging from 30 days to 180 days. Typically, the longer you are able to wait, the lower your premium will be. However, a policy with a 30-day waiting period could actually take as long as 90 days before it begins paying benefits (retroactive to the 31st day after onset of your disability). That's because your disability will need to be verified, as will your salary at the time you became disabled.

Observation: *My husband's disability policy had a 30-day waiting period. I submitted the claim for his benefits less than a month after he entered the hospital. We received the first check about 80 days after he was hospitalized—covering only the first four weeks of benefits. The second check, covering three more weeks, arrived on the 85th day. The third check, covering another two weeks, arrived on the 90th day. Thereafter, weekly payments, covering the preceding week, arrived like clockwork.*

Individual Disability Insurance: Key Points

As we've said, individual disability insurance policies generally are more expensive than group insurance. But there are advantages. You can select the amount of the benefit, how soon after a disability you'll begin receiving it and how long you will continue to get it. The policy can cover you wherever you move or work. And because you're buying the policy with after-tax dollars, the entire benefit is tax free. This means you need enough to match only your take-home pay, not your full income.

Caution: *Many of the policies sold in conjunction with credit cards (guaranteeing to pay your minimum monthly payment if you are disabled), with auto and bank loans (such as mortgage disability income insurance) or through telemarketing or mass mailings tend to be low quality and will not provide much relief in the*

State-Sponsored Disability Programs

As of this writing, only five states—California, Hawaii, New Jersey, New York and Rhode Island—sponsor disability programs for residents. These programs are generally short term and have low benefit ceilings. In California, for example, the maximum benefit in 1997 was $336 per week for 52 weeks.

You may want to check with your state to determine what, if any, benefits are available and the eligibility requirements. However, with regard to planning your financial safety net, keep in mind that these programs would offset only a small portion of the economic loss you want to avoid.

event of disability. Your best bet is to calculate your assets and liabilities as we recommended previously, so you can purchase sufficient coverage to keep you from defaulting on your credit cards and loans. Then go with a well-known, well-rated insurance company that has a good track record with its disability policies.

To find out which companies offer individual disability income insurance, you may wish to obtain the free directory from the Health Insurance Association of America. Be aware, however, that the directory contains only companies that are members of HIAA. Its Web address is http://www.hiaa.org, or you can call the HIAA's Insurance Education Program at (202) 824-1673.

You should also inquire as to whether disability insurance is available through your union or professional association. The premiums are often lower than if you purchase an individual policy.

If you are eligible, you can buy individual disability income insurance that will pay benefits anywhere from two years to as long as you live. In general, the longer the maximum benefit period, the higher the cost. You should buy coverage so that benefits will continue until you can begin receiving retirement income.

If your employer offers a medical disability retirement option, you may need coverage for only two to five years: basically, the period until your retirement application is processed and approved. A five-year benefit period would make sense, for example, if your disability retirement pay is 50 percent of your average annual earnings for the previous three years. However, if your disability retirement income would be only a small fraction of your original salary (which could be the case if you were employed only a short time), you may need a policy that pays benefits for the rest of your life.

Caution: *If you are age 50 or older and you buy disability insurance with lifetime benefits, the insurance company might reduce your monthly benefit by as much as 50 percent when you reach age 65.* However, if you buy the same policy before age 50, the insurance company may continue paying the full benefit even after you're 65.

Choose a policy with an appropriate waiting period. Recognize that it may take 30 days or more to

Key Policy Terms

When comparing disability insurance policies, keep in mind the following terms:

Own occupation: This definition of disability means that you cannot do your job, even if you can do something else.

Residual disability: This allows you to work at your job part time and still receive a portion of your benefit.

Inflation protection: Once you are disabled, your benefits will increase along with inflation.

Guaranteed renewable: The insurance company can never cancel your policy but can raise the premiums for the general class in which you are a member.

Optionally renewable: The insurance company can extend your policy at each premium due date, but it is not required to do so.

Noncancelable: This prevents the insurance company from changing your policy or premium.

Make sure you understand how a policy defines "disability." The most liberal definitions—covering the inability to perform your current job—are the most desirable but also the most expensive. Consider buying a policy where you have an "own occupation" definition of disability for the first two to three years and a reasonable definition of disability for the duration of the disability.

Caution: *Some policies require that a person be confined to a hospital in order to collect disability benefits. Steer clear of policies like this. Likewise, avoid policies that will not pay benefits unless you cannot perform* ***any*** *occupation.*

complete the paperwork for filing your claim. A typical claim involves three parts: one for you to fill out, one for your employer to fill out (even if you bought the policy yourself) and one for your physician to fill out. If you're in the hospital, someone else will need to file the claim for you, which could add even more time to the process—particularly if a copy of your insurance policy isn't readily at hand *(see Section 3).*

➤ **Recommendation:** *Select a waiting period that's three months less than the longest waiting period your finances will allow. That way, if your claim takes two or three months to process, you won't run into financial difficulties before you receive the first check. Also, you may discover that the extra benefits come in handy for meeting the expenses often incurred during the first few weeks or months of an emergency, such as calling out-of-state relatives, obtaining and photocopying the records you need for filing your claim and consulting with a lawyer. If you're lucky enough not to need the extra financial cushion, then use the insurance benefits to replace some of the money you took out of your emergency fund.*

If possible, choose a policy that waives payment of premiums during the time you're receiving benefits under the policy. Some policies also offer a **Social Security rider,** which pays you extra income if you are disabled and have been turned down by Social Security for disability insurance benefits (7 out of 10 applications are initially refused).

Some individual disability income policies offer riders that provide money to support your children's education if you are disabled. Others offer a **savings supplement option,** which allows you to protect up to an additional 10 percent of monthly earnings to compensate for lost savings opportunities as a result of a long-term disability.

There may also be a **future-adjustment option,** which enables you to increase your individual coverage if your salary increases or if your group long-term disability coverage is lost or reduced as a result of changes in employment or in employer-provided benefits.

Specialized Disability Insurance for Business Owners

If you own a business, you may want to look into the following specialized disability insurance policies.

Business overhead expense

This type of insurance pays your eligible business expenses in the event you are disabled. Typically, eligible expenses include any regular expense, normally incurred in the conduct of your business or profession, which requires a cash payment and is considered tax deductible by the IRS. The policy generally has a short elimination (waiting) period and a one- to two-year benefit period, which should give you enough time to determine whether your disability will force you to sell the business. If you have high fixed expenses, you should consider purchasing this insurance.

Disability buyout

If one of your partners/shareholders becomes permanently disabled, it may become necessary to buy out his interest. However, your business may already be struggling as a result of that individual's disability, so buying him out at that point could financially strain your firm. A disability buyout policy can provide the money (either in a lump sum or installments) to purchase the interest of the disabled partner/shareholder.

Disability key-man (employee)

If a key employee becomes disabled, your first reaction may be to continue paying that individual. However, in the absence of a Qualified Sick Pay Plan, adopted prior to an employee's disability, any wages you voluntarily pay (and FICA contributions) to a disabled employee or stockholder-employee are not considered tax-deductible business expenses by the IRS. If you want to provide continuing income to a key employee, without having your business take a financial hit, consider buying this type of policy.

While this can be a good purchase, keep in mind that when you exercise this option, it may be priced at your attained age, not your age at original issue. Also, you might not be able to exercise this option if you are disabled.

Tips on Shopping for Disability Insurance

When comparing policies, you should ask the following questions:

✔ **Definition of "disability"**

—Are education, experience and past earnings taken into account in determining what you can reasonably be expected to do?
—Does the policy provide an "own occupation" or "any occupation" definition for "disability"?

✔ **Partial or residual disability**

—Are benefits provided when your medical condition allows you to perform only a portion of your duties? (This may also be called **income replacement** because the amount of the payout depends on how much income you lose.)
—Is this benefit payable only when preceded by a period of total disability?

✔ **Cost of living adjustment**

—Is a COLA available to increase benefit payouts subsequent to disability and protect you against inflation? (The younger you are when the policy is issued, the more important this benefit may be.)

✔ **Renewability**

—Is the policy noncancelable and guaranteed renewable until you reach age 65?

Note: Some industry experts say insurance companies will be getting away from noncancelable (fixed-premium) policies within the next five years. Most policies will be guaranteed renewable, but premiums will be allowed to change. If you cannot afford a fixed-premium policy, you should consider a step-rated one, which is almost always cheaper initially. With a step-rated policy, your premiums increase as you age, generally in five-year increments, but sometimes annually. If you don't need disability insurance for more than, say, 10 years, the step-rated policy could be a very good buy.

✔ **Waiting or elimination periods**

—Are they proper for your circumstances?

✔ **Benefit period**

—How long will the policy pay you benefits? (The younger you are when the policy is issued, the more important it is to have a long—even lifetime—benefit period. A career-ending disability when you're in your 30s, for example, will significantly lower your pension benefits, other assets and even Social Security benefits.)

Many disability insurance policies offer a provision under which you can receive a refund of seven or eight years' worth of premiums if you go 10 years without a disability. If, however, you become disabled, any future return of premiums will be reduced by any disability benefits paid. This option is very expensive and can boost the price of the policy by as much as 50 percent. You're probably better off investing the amount you'd pay for this option.

Another provision to be wary of is one that pays lifetime benefits if you are injured in an accident but pays benefits only to age 65 for a disabling illness. From a financial perspective, you are just as badly affected by a medical condition as by an accident. It does not make sense, therefore, to try to get a better accident benefit than illness benefit.

POTENTIAL DIFFICULTIES IN OBTAINING DISABILITY INSURANCE

Purchasing individual disability income insurance may not be easy. It's important to apply for it while you're in good health. If you wait until you have a medical problem, you may still be able to get coverage—but it may exclude coverage for your particular condition or cost extra because of your health history.

Premiums are usually determined on the basis of your age, sex and occupation. The older you are, the greater your risk of disability and, therefore, the more costly the insurance. Women tend to have more claims, so they are usually charged higher premiums than men.

Worse yet, some insurance companies won't cover you if they deem your occupation too risky. You may be surprised to know that ineligible occupations can include a butler, composer/songwriter, makeup artist, private music teacher, nanny, televangelist and valet. *(See the list on page 34.)*

If you can describe your job differently from how it appears on an insurance company's list of ineligible occupations (such as "preacher" instead of "televangelist"), you might be able to get insurance. However, the insurance company could later contend that you falsified your application and deny your claim—leaving you without insurance and forcing you to eat the cost of all the premiums you've paid. So before you attempt to play word games with the underwriters, remember that just because one insurance company won't insure your occupation, another company may. Alternatively, you may find a professional association that offers a disability insurance benefit to people in the same occupation as yours.

DISABILITY INCOME FROM MORE THAN ONE SOURCE

Some insurance experts recommend buying as much disability income insurance as you are eligible for and can afford. There are a number of reasons you might want to follow this advice. First, you can never have too much tax-free income, particularly if you're able to invest some of it in a mutual fund or other vehicle where the earnings have tax-deferred status. Second, there's no guarantee that your injury or medical condition will be covered by workers' comp or Social Security. Third, if you have a group disability policy, the benefits you receive are taxable—effectively reducing your benefit to only 30 percent to 40 percent of your take-home pay, which probably is not enough to keep the wolf from the door.

By contrast, some insurance experts recommend that you not pay the extra expense of getting 100 percent income replacement. One reason is that you don't get a tax deduction on your premiums, which could be a couple thousand dollars a year if you're a high-earner. Second, if your policy has a **coordination of benefits** or **integration of benefits provision**, you won't receive all the benefits you've paid for in the event you end up getting disability income from other sources (such as workers' comp, Social Security, other group or individual disability or, in some cases, sick pay).

A coordination of benefits provision allows the insurance company to deduct all, or a percentage of, the other benefits you receive from the amount it would ordinarily pay you. Thus, if your policy benefit is $2,000 a month and you receive $1,200 a month in disability income from Social Security, the insurance company will pay you only $800 a month—even though you've paid premiums based on receiving $2,000 a month.

Workers' comp, Social Security

Before you decide which approach is best, you should be aware that workers' comp and Social Security disability benefits cover only a minimal amount of your earnings, especially for a permanent injury. In terms of lifetime earnings, you may end up receiving only about 20 cents on the dollar. Moreover, some of these benefits may be taxable as ordinary income.

Workers' compensation benefits generally are not taxable. However, if you return to work after qualifying for workers' comp, any payments you continue to receive while assigned to light duties are taxable. Similarly, if part of your workers' compensation reduces the amount of Social Security benefits you receive, that part is considered Social Security benefits and may be taxable.

Federal workers are covered under the Federal Employees' Compensation Act (FECA), the government's version of workers' comp. FECA benefits are not taxable if they are paid because of a work-related injury or sickness. However, payments received as "continuation of pay" for up to 45 days while a claim is being decided are taxable. Likewise, pay received for sick leave while a claim is being processed is taxable.

Some people who get **Social Security disability benefits** have to pay taxes on a certain percentage of the benefits. If you file a federal tax return as an individual and your "combined income" is between $25,000 and $34,000, you may have to pay taxes on 50 percent of your Social Security benefits. (The Social Security Administration defines "combined income" as the sum of your adjusted gross income plus nontaxable interest plus one-half of your Social Security benefits.) If your combined income is above $34,000, up to 85 percent of your Social Security benefits is subject to income tax. If you file a joint return, you may have to pay taxes on 50 percent of your Social Security disability benefits if you and your spouse have a combined income between $32,000 and $44,000. If your combined income is more than $44,000, up to 85 percent of your Social Security benefits are subject to income tax.

LONG-TERM-CARE INSURANCE: THE SECOND HALF OF THE EQUATION

Long-term-care policies (LTCs) cover medical care, nursing care and other assistance you might need if a chronic illness or disability leaves you unable to care for yourself for an extended time. These services generally are not covered by other health insurance. You may receive long-term care in a nursing home or in your own home. In general, three types of care are associated with long-term care:

- **Skilled nursing care:** for medical conditions that require care by skilled medical personnel, such as registered nurses or professional therapists. This care, available 24 hours a day, is ordered by a physician and involves a treatment plan.

(Continued on page 36)

Occupations Ineligible for Disability Insurance

If your occupation is listed here, some insurance companies may refuse to issue you an individual disabil insurance policy. The following list of ineligible occupations was compiled by The Guardian Life Insuranc Company of America.

Actor/Actress
Aerobics/Exercise Instructor
Aesthetician
Air Evacuation Personnel
Air Traffic Controller
Aircraft Pilot
Algologist [person who studies algae]
Ambulance Driver
Antenna or Tower Worker
Appliance Repairer
Arbitrageur
Armored Car Driver/Worker
Asbestos Remover/Pipe Wrapper
Asphalt Worker
Assembly Line Worker
Athlete (pro or semi-pro)
Attendant (parking)
Attendant (hospital, nursing home)
Auto Body Shop Employee

Baggage Handler
Bail Bondsman/Employee
Bank Guard/Watchman
Bar/Nightclub Owner
Bar/Nightclub Worker
Barber
Bartender
Beautician
Bellboy/Doorman
Billboard Worker
Blacksmith
Body Shop Employee
Bodyguard
Bridge Worker
Building Mgr./Supervisor
Busboy
Bus Driver
Butler

Caisson Worker
Camp Counselor
Car Wash Employee
Carpet Installer/Cleaner
Chauffeur
Check-Cashing Employee
Chimney Cleaner
Commodities Broker/Trader (on floor)
Composer/Songwriter
Concrete/Cement Worker
Convenience Store Worker
Cook
Cosmetologist
Counter Worker
Crane/Derrick/Hoist Operator
Crop Duster
Custodian

Dairy Worker
Dance Instructor
Dancer
Day Care Worker
Dealer (gambling industry)
Deli Worker
Delivery Person
Demolition Worker
Diver
Diving Instructor
Dock Worker
Domestic Service Worker
Door-to-Door Salesperson
Doorman
Driver (any vehicle)
Dyer/Bleacher

Electrologist
Electroplater
Elevator Operator
Engineer (train, caisson, experimental flying, underwater)
Explosives Worker
Exterminator

Factory Worker
Farm/Ranch Employee
Fast-Food Worker
Firefighter
Firewood Cutting/Delivery
Fisherman
Fishing Boat Owner or Officer/Crew
Flight Attendant
Flight Instructor
Floor Broker (securities)
Food-Processing Worker
Foreman (oil field)
Forklift Operator
Freight Handler
Futures Broker/Trader (on floor)

Garbage Collector
Guard

Hairdresser
Harbor/Dock Master
Harbor Pilot
Hazardous-Waste Worker

Health Club/Pool/Spa Worker
Heavy-Equipment Operator
Home Health Care Worker
Hospital Orderly
Housekeeper/Maid

Instructor (aerobics, martial arts, skating, skiing, etc.)

Janitor
Junk Dealer/Owner/Yard Worker

Kennel Owner/Worker
Kitchen Worker

Laborer
Laundry Worker
Law Enforcement Officer
Lineman (overhead wires)
Logging Worker
Longshoreman

Maid
Maintenance (cleaning)
Makeup Artist
Manicurist
Marina Worker
Market Maker (securities, trading own account)
Martial Arts Instructor
Masseuse
Matron
Military (active duty)
Mine Worker
Model
Music Teacher (private lessons)
Musician (if not full-time salaried)

Nanny
Newsstand Owner/Worker
Nightclub Owner or Mgr./Employee
Nuclear Energy Worker
Nurse (private duty, any degree)
Nurse's Aide

Office Temporary Worker
Offshore Worker
Options Broker/Trader (on floor)
Orderly

Packing/Slaughterhouse Worker or Supervisor
Parts (delivery)
Party/Charter Boat Captain/Crew
Photographer (freelance)
Pilot
Pipeline Worker
Pit Boss (gambling industry)
Pit Broker (securities)
Pizza Parlor Worker
Police Officer
Position Trader (securities)
Postal Service Employee
Prison Worker
Private Detective

Quarry Worker

Railroad Worker
Refinery Worker
Repo Person (of cars, etc.)
Roofer
Route Salesperson
Runner/Delivery Person or Messenger

Sandblaster
Sanitation Supervisor/Worker
Sawmill Worker
Screenwriter (freelance)
Scuba Instructor
Sculptor
Security Person
Service Station Employee
Sewage Supervisor/Worker
Shoemaker/Repairer
Shoe Shiner
Shop/Boat Crew
Singer
Skating Instructor
Skiing Instructor
Slaughterhouse Worker
Stable Owner/Worker
Steeplejack
Superintendent (apartment building)

Telephone Solicitor
Televangelist
Timber Cruiser
Trader (securities)
Tree Sprayer
Tree Surgeon
Truck Driver
Tunnel Worker

Unskilled Worker

Valet
Visiting Nurse

Waiter/Waitress
Warehouse Worker
Watchman
Weightlifting Instructor/Trainer
Window Washer
Woods Worker (lumberjack)
Writer (freelance)

(Continued from page 33)

- **Intermediate nursing care:** for stable conditions that require daily, but not 24-hour nursing supervision. Such care is ordered by a physician and supervised by registered nurses.
- **Custodial care:** for persons needing help performing activities of daily living (ADLs), such as bathing, eating and dressing. Sometimes called personal care, it is usually provided by people without medical skills.
  Note: If you hire a personal aide, rather than a home health care worker, to provide custodial care, the cost may be deductible as a "dependent care" expense, but you'll have to pay Social Security and other employment taxes.

Long-term care may be provided in settings other than a nursing home or your own home, including the following:

Assisted-living facilities: These provide supportive, personal or nursing services in an apartment-like setting. Generally, they must be certified or registered with the state.

Adult day care: This is a nonresidential, structured program designed to meet the health, social and other support needs of functionally impaired adults.

Respite care: This service provides personal care and supervision for a functionally impaired individual in order to give a family member or other primary caregiver temporary relief from caregiving duties. Usually, respite care services are provided in the impaired individual's home but may sometimes be in a nursing home.

Hospice care: This is a specially designed package of social and medical services that provide pain relief, symptom management and supportive services to terminally ill people and their families.

Most LTC policies pay a fixed amount—typically $40 to $200 a day—for care you receive in a nursing home. The daily benefit for at-home care is usually half the benefit for nursing home care. Because the per-day benefit you buy today may be inadequate to cover higher costs in the future, most policies offer an **inflation adjustment feature**.

As with any insurance, the amount of coverage you need depends on your circumstances. At a minimum, the coverage should be sufficient to protect your assets. For example, if you receive monthly retirement income of $2,500 and a nursing home costs $5,500 monthly, your LTC insurance benefit should be at least $3,000 to cover the difference. If you have dependents, you need to purchase enough coverage to protect both your income and your assets. You can reduce the size of your premiums by selecting a longer waiting period, higher deductible or shorter benefit period or by forgoing inflation protection. Elder law attorneys frequently suggest that children pay the premiums, in whole or in part, for their parents' LTC insurance as a sort of "inheritance protection."

In general, the younger you are when applying for LTC insurance, the lower your premiums will be. Rates increase substantially at age 60 and again after age 65. After purchase, the premiums remain the same. Although most financial planners recommend that long-term-care insurance be purchased in your late 50s or early 60s, when premiums are still relatively affordable and you probably are still healthy enough to be insurable, you should seriously consider buying LTC insurance as soon as you can. In fact, the Health Insurance Portability and Accountability Act of 1996 *(see page 37)* provides some incentives to purchase LTC insurance at an earlier age.

Observation: *A catastrophic injury or illness can strike at any age.* ***In fact, 43 percent of those needing long-term care today are under age 65.*** *I bought LTC insurance in 1994 for my* *husband (then age 46) and myself (then age 39). Including the inflation-adjustment rider, among other benefits, the annual premium for my husband is only $612.48 for $3,000 worth of monthly nursing home coverage ($1,500 for home health care), while mine is just $471.03 for the same amount of coverage. Even after my husband's stroke, his premiums did not increase.*

LTC provisions of the Health Insurance Act

Since passage of the Health Insurance Portability and Accountability Act, insurers are able to market tax-favored LTC insurance policies to protect against individuals becoming "chronically ill." There are several requirements that LTC policies (and the insurers) must meet to be treated as Qualified Long-Term-Care Insurance Contracts. Policies in existence prior to Jan. 1, 1997, are grandfathered, as long as they meet whatever long-term-care requirements your state may have.

Special tax advantages arise because these qualified contracts will be treated as if they were health insurance policies. This means that the benefits paid for such policies can be received tax free (within certain limits, discussed below). Further, the premiums paid by your employer for your contract can be deducted from taxes and won't be included in your income.

If you buy an individual qualified LTC contract, some or all of the premiums may qualify for an individual tax deduction (you have to itemize deductions to use this tax break), and the benefits (up to $175 a day) you receive will be tax free.

If you're self-employed, you can write off a percentage of your premium as a business expense (40 percent this year, gradually rising to 100 percent by 2007). Formerly, these tax breaks were not available if you were covered (or eligible to be covered) under another health insurance policy—for example, as a dependent on your spouse's plan.

The amount of premiums qualifying for favorable tax treatment varies according to your age. If you are 40 or younger, the annual premiums that can be deducted may not exceed $200 per year. This figure goes up by 10-year age brackets, to $375 per year for people ages 41 to 50; $750 for ages 51 to 60; $2,000 for ages 61 to 70; and $2,500 for individuals older than 70. (These limits will rise with inflation.) The insurance company will issue you a 1099 form for the amount of benefits paid each year.

You may not purchase a Qualified Long-Term-Care Insurance Contract through a cafeteria plan; therefore, the premiums may not be reimbursed through flexible spending accounts (FSAs). However, you may use Medical Savings Accounts (*discussed on page 20*) to pay for the contract's premiums and services.

LTC expenses qualify for the tax deduction if:

- You, your spouse or a dependent is expected to be "chronically ill" for at least 90 days, as determined by a doctor, registered nurse or licensed social worker.
- The expenses are part of a specified treatment plan (also called "plan of care").
- The expenses aren't reimbursed by insurance.
- The services are not performed by a relative, unless that relative is licensed to do so.
- You are not also taking the dependent-care credit on your tax return.

Medicare: Not a good substitute for LTC insurance

Contrary to what many believe, Medicare doesn't come close to providing the amount of coverage you get with long-term-care insurance. If you participate in the Medicare program (that is, you are at least 65 years old or, if younger than 65, have been eligible for Social Security disability benefits for 24 months), Medicare might pay for some of your LTC expenses—but don't count on it. For additional coverage, Medicare recipients usually purchase supplemental Medigap policies, but even these do not fully cover long-term care. Moreover, if you are younger than 65 and on Social Security disability, you might not even be able to buy—or afford—adequate Medigap insurance.

If Medicare approves a nursing home stay, the program pays in full for up to 20 days of skilled nursing care in a Medicare-certified facility. However, Medicare will pay only if your nursing home stay follows three days' hospitalization and you enter a Medicare-certified nursing home within 30 days after hospital discharge. From the 21st to the 100th day, Medicare pays part of the cost. Beyond the 100th day, it pays nothing. Moreover, it does not cover intermediate or custodial care, or prolonged home health care.

Caution: *Few people actually receive 100 days of Medicare nursing home coverage.* The average number of days Medicare pays for is less than 30. Most nursing home stays aren't covered by Medicare at all—because many nursing homes do not participate in the Medicare program (Medicare pays too little to make it worth their while) and because Medicare defines "skilled care" in very restrictive terms.

As for home health care, Medicare covers only those expenses it considers "medically necessary" (defined very narrowly) and that meet certain other criteria. For example:

- The care must include part-time skilled nursing care, physical therapy or speech therapy.
- You must be confined to home.
- The doctor must set up a home health treatment plan.
- The home health agency providing services must participate in Medicare.

Note: Most home health care visits do not meet Medicare's definition of "medically necessary" care. Therefore, Medicare will not pay for them.

Who should buy LTC insurance?

If your annual income is modest—say, under $15,000—and your assets are small, financial planners usually recommend that you not buy long-term-care insurance. The premiums can eat up a sizable portion of your assets, significantly reducing your standard of living, particularly if you are elderly. Besides, if you enter a nursing home and run through your own resources, Medicaid will likely pick up the bill. (Remember, though, that Medicaid will look back at least three years to make sure you didn't transfer assets at less than fair market value. Also, after you die, Medicaid may put a lien on your estate to recover the amount of benefits it paid on your behalf.)

The United Seniors Health Cooperative, a nonprofit consumer organization, offers the following guidelines to use in deciding whether to buy LTC insurance:

✔ If you have more than $75,000 in assets (not counting your house and car) for every person in the household, long-term-care insurance will enable you to leave at least part of those assets to your heirs.

✔ If your annual income is $30,000 or more for every person in the household, you shouldn't have trouble affording the premiums for LTC insurance.

✔ If your premiums will cost less than 10 percent of your income, long-term-care insurance is a sound investment.

✔ If you could still afford to buy the policy if its cost went up by as much as 30 percent, you should consider getting it.

If you and your spouse are in equally good health but can afford to buy only one policy, generally the policy should cover the wife, not the husband. That's because women tend to live longer and hence are more subject to the types of disease, like Alzheimer's, that require long-term care.

Other ways to pay for long-term care

If you cannot afford an LTC policy at all, you may want to consider a nursing-home-only insurance policy or home-health-care-only policy. Of the two, it's advisable to purchase the nursing home coverage—unless you have relatives who will help provide care in your home or theirs.

Another way to cover long-term-care expenses is through a rider attached to a life insurance policy. In that case, your monthly benefit will typically be based on a percentage of the life insurance amount. For example, on a $100,000 policy, a 2 percent benefit will give you $2,000 a month for covered nursing home care. A monthly benefit for home health care, covered under the rider, is usually half the nursing home benefit.

Caution: *Long-term-care benefits under life insurance riders are directly tied to the amount of life insurance in force.* Such benefits will be reduced by any loans or withdrawals you have taken against the policy. Using the long-term-care benefits will also reduce the life insurance coverage under the policy.

A long-term-care rider has a separate insurance charge, which usually increases each year in a manner similar to the cost of the life insurance under the basic poli-

How a Viatical Settlement Works

To qualify as a "viator," you must be diagnosed with a terminal illness. For your life insurance policy to be eligible for a viatical settlement, you must have the option to change the right of ownership or freely assign coverage. Any person listed as a beneficiary must sign a release and waive all current and future rights to the proceeds from your policy.

Typically, viatical settlement providers do not charge the viator any fee, and you may receive your settlement as soon as three to five weeks after submitting your application. However, if your policy is less than two years old and still in its "contestability" period (that is, the insurance company could find some fault with you or your policy and cancel it), you may not be able to get a viatical settlement provider to do business with you.

The viatical settlement provider will review your medical records and evaluate your policy terms to determine a maximum selling price for your policy. Essentially, the viatical settlement provider will offer to sell your policy to people hoping to get very high returns on their investments. (In other words, the investor's profit depends on your dying sooner, rather than later. For example, if the investor buys a $100,000 policy for $55,000 and you die before the investor has had to pay any premiums to keep the policy in force, the return on the investment is $45,000, or nearly 82 percent.)

In most cases, your responsibility for future premiums on your policy ends with its sale. However, in the case of Federal Employees' Government Life Insurance (FEGLI), federal employees and annuitants are required by the government to continue paying the premiums, even after assigning their coverage.

Caution: *A viatical settlement could adversely affect your qualification status for income-based federal or state financial assistance.*

cy. The annual charge for the rider will not exceed the maximum guaranteed cost and will normally be less.

If you have a cash-value life insurance policy (also called permanent life or universal life), you may be able to take out money to help pay for your long-term-care needs. You can do so either through preferred loans (often at or near an effective interest rate of 0 percent) taken against the cash value of the policy or partial withdrawals of your original basis, or both. If done carefully (you should consult professional advisers), the money you take out may even be tax free.

Alternatively, you may decide to convert your life insurance benefits into tax-free "living benefits," under the "Accelerated Death Benefits" ("viatical settlements") provisions of the Health Insurance Portability and Accountability Act of 1996. As of Jan. 1, 1997, any amount received under a life insurance contract on the life of a terminally ill or chronically ill insured is treated as an amount paid by reason of the insured's death and, therefore, is not taxable. This holds true, too, for any amount you receive (typically between 55 percent and 85 percent of the face value) from selling or assigning your life insurance policy to someone else (usually done through a viatical settlement provider). (*See box on page 39.*)

Insurance Policies to Avoid

Some policies are simply not worth the premiums. Unfortunately, a small number of insurance agents target the elderly and rural residents, who can least afford these types of insurance.

❑ **Cancer Insurance:** This type of policy pays only if you get cancer. Usually the coverage is totally inadequate, paying a maximum benefit of $250,000.

❑ **Other Dread-Disease Insurance:** These policies pay covered charges for specified diseases, such as poliomyelitis, tetanus, encephalitis, tularemia, meningitis, diphtheria, rabies, psittacosis, brucellosis, typhoid fever, cholera, toxic shock syndrome, Reye's syndrome and legionellosis. Again, the coverage usually is totally inadequate, typically paying a lifetime benefit of $100,000.

❑ **Hospital Income (or Indemnity) Insurance:** This insurance pays you between $50 and $350 for each day you are in the hospital. The cash benefit is intended to help you pay for uninsured medical expenses. However, only certain types of hospitalization are covered (for example, only an accident or a covered sickness). If you have a good health insurance policy, you probably won't need the extra cash—particularly if you also have a disability insurance policy.

As a last-ditch method of paying for long-term care, some elderly homeowners take out a **reverse mortgage**. Financial advisers generally do not recommend this. Hidden fees can wipe out not only any proceeds you or your heirs receive from the sale of your home but also a significant portion of any other assets you may have. Nevertheless, if you haven't planned well for long-term care, this is an option you should consider.

A reverse mortgage is a way of borrowing against the equity you have in your home. You can get a lump sum, line of credit or monthly payments. As a loan, the money you receive is not taxable. However, if monthly payments are not spent in the month received, the remaining amount will be counted as a resource for Supplemental Security Income and Medicaid eligibility purposes.

No repayment is normally required for as long as you live in the house. The interest is simply added as a mortgage to the property, which is then paid off when you die. The interest rate currently is about 6 percent to 8 percent.

Caution: *If you decide to move, you'll have to pay off the reverse mortgage plus interest and fees. This is where people have run into a lot of trouble.*

Currently, about 125 lenders offer reverse mortgages to homeowners over age 62. The amount they offer can vary as much as $30,000, so it's vitally important to shop around. The four major reverse-mortgage programs available are the "Home Equity Conversion Plan," which is insured by the Department of Housing and Urban Development; the "Household" program by Household Bank (not available in all states); TransAmerica's "HomeFirst Plan" (not available in all states); and Fannie Mae's "HomeKeeper Mortgage."

➤ **Recommendation:** *Do business only with a lender that has the "seal of approval" of the nonprofit National Center for Home Equity Conversion (NCHEC). These lenders offer a unique NCHEC software program that compares the major loans available to you. There also are NCHEC-approved counselors who agree to abide by a code of conduct. For a list of NCHEC-approved lenders and counselors, write to NCHEC Preferred, Room 115, 7373 147th St., Apple Valley, MN 55124.*

How to compare LTC policies

First, you should look at how the policy pays benefits. For example, some policies pay a fixed amount for each day you are confined in a nursing home, regardless of the actual cost of care. Other policies pay according to the provider's actual charges, up to a fixed daily amount or a percentage of the charges.

You should also examine the length of time benefits will be paid. Benefits may last for the rest of your lifetime or only one year. In general, plans that provide payments for longer periods of time are more expensive. On the other hand, you may not be able to increase the benefit period at a later date without proving insurability.

Policies frequently limit benefits to certain services provided by specific types of facilities or agencies. For example, services provided in the home may be limited to those provided by a licensed home health agency. Other types of personal care or help with household chores may not be covered. Check each policy to see exactly what's covered and whether the services are what you need and want.

You should determine whether premium payments are based on "issue age" or "attained age." Issue age means that you pay a level premium determined by your age when you bought the policy. Attained-age premiums automatically increase as you get older. Some policies limit premium payments to a given period of time, such as 10 or 20 years.

Long-term-care policies pay benefits based on certain "triggers," called activities of daily living (ADLs). Most policies base benefits on six specific ADLs and pay benefits when you require assistance to perform at least three of the ADLs or have a cognitive impairment.

If you're already sick or under a doctor's care for a particular condition when you buy an LTC policy, you may not be eligible for benefits for that condition until a certain period has passed. Your state may have a limit on how long this waiting period for a pre-existing condition can last. For example, Wisconsin has a six-month limit.

Aside from the waiting period for pre-existing conditions, LTC policies frequently have an elimination period before they start paying benefits. Usually, the longer the period—typically no more than 365 days—the lower the premium. Be aware, though, that

Long-Term-Care Insurance Checklist

This checklist can be used to compare the costs and benefits of policies you are considering.

Name and address of insurance company: ______________________

Phone number: ______________________

Name and address of agent: ______________________

Phone number: ______________________

Type of Care Covered

Institutional Care	**Daily Benefit**	**Length of Benefit**	**Limitations**
Nursing Home	$______	______	______
Assisted-Living Facility	$______	______	______
Hospice Facility	$______	______	______
Bed Reservation Guarantee			

Community-Based Care	**Daily Benefit**	**Length of Benefit**	**Limitations**
Home Health Care	$______	______	______
Adult Day Care	$______	______	______
Respite Care	$______	______	______
Hospice	$______	______	______
Other	$______	______	______

Elimination Period

Per Occurrence

Per Lifetime

Waiting Period for Pre-existing Conditions

Premium Payment Period

Attained Age (premiums increase as you age)

Issue Age (premiums won't rise merely because you get older)

Lifetime or Period-Specific

Policy Exclusions and Limitations

Waiver of Premium

Inflation Protection

Nonforfeiture Benefits

(If you discontinue coverage, a nonforfeiture benefit allows you to recoup a portion of your payments or continue coverage at a lower level.)

Cost of Policy

Basic Policy	$______
Inflation Protection	$______
Nonforfeiture Benefits	$______
Additional Benefits	$______

the longer the elimination period, the less chance you will have to collect benefits. Also, pay close attention to policy exclusions. The most common are for mental and nervous disorders, pre-existing conditions, care received outside the United States and care needed for a self-inflicted injury.

Don't Keep Your Spouse in the Dark

3

After my husband had been in intensive care for two and a half weeks, the attending physician would say only that the stroke had caused some brain damage. No prognosis was forthcoming. At the time, John was on life support, and there were days he didn't recognize me. It was too late to write the wills we'd talked about or our "advance medical directives" telling when it would be OK to "pull the plug." Of more immediate concern, I didn't know how I would deposit John's disability income checks when they arrived since I didn't have his "power of attorney." I realized I'd better see a lawyer—fast.

If the Ceiling Fell on You Right Now . . .

Would someone be able to step into your shoes if you were suddenly blinded, paralyzed or rendered unconscious? Does that person know your insurance policy ID number? What medications you're taking? Who your doctor is? Does someone at work know your password for retrieving your voice mail or logging onto your computer? Would there be anyone to feed your dog, take your car for inspection, file your tax return or get your suits back from the dry cleaner?

At a minimum, there are two things you need to do—in advance of an emergency—to keep things running smoothly if you're out of commission. The first is to appoint someone to be your **attorney in fact**, giving that person legal authority to conduct your personal, medical and business affairs. The second is to compile an instruction kit or "Answers Book," telling your attorney in fact where every record is and, if necessary, what to do with it. *You should do both of these things right now.* Once you're injured or ill, you may not be capable of telling anyone anything.

You Don't Have to Be a Lawyer . . .

When you go out of town, a friend or a neighbor might routinely take in your mail, mow your lawn or even use a spare key to water the plants in your living room. Technically speaking, the person doing these favors for you would be guilty of interfering with the U.S. mail, trespassing and conversion—unless you've given that person written permission to do those tasks for you. The piece of paper giving such authorization to that individual is what's known as a **power of attorney**.

Of course, people usually don't get into legal trouble for doing simple chores for friends or neighbors without the formality of a power of attorney. In most cases, these little favors don't come to other people's attention, so nobody has reason to be concerned. Also, people are inclined to assume that whoever is helping out has permission to do so.

Nevertheless, your tacit or verbal permission has its limits. A banker, for one, isn't going to let someone into your safe deposit box merely on that person's (or even your) say-so. When you need more than casual help with your financial, medical or personal affairs, a power of attorney is a must.

Granting a power of attorney

By granting someone power of attorney, you transfer responsibility for managing virtually every aspect of your life—whether it be running your business or your household, making decisions about your medical care, investing your retirement savings or almost any decision-making activity you can name. In legal jargon, you are the **grantor** of the power of attorney, and the recipient of your power of attorney is your **attorney in fact** (sometimes called **attorney in law and in fact**).

You can give as much or as little responsibility (or power of attorney) to as many people as you deem necessary. For example, you can give power of attorney to (1) your spouse to make your medical decisions, (2) your financial planner or lawyer to handle your financial affairs and (3) your business partner to keep the company running.

You can even give **joint power of attorney** to two or more people, specifying that they can act only in concert. For example, you might give joint power of attorney to both your parents or all your children, stating that they must be in agreement before they can act on your behalf. Alternatively, your joint power of attorney could specify that any of the named parties may act singly. For example, you might give joint power of attorney to your spouse and your daughter, with the understanding that if your spouse becomes ill or incapacitated, your daughter will take over as attorney in fact.

Observation: *Some people (an elderly parent, a spouse, a business partner) may feel that their independence is threatened by signing a power of attorney. Consider having reciprocal powers of attorney prepared, naming you and another person as each other's attorney in fact. This might alleviate the concern that one of you is taking advantage of the other.*

The most important factors to consider when choosing your attorney in fact are:

❑ **Do you trust this individual?** If you have any concerns about the person's honesty or reliability, then don't give him your power of attorney.

❑ **Is this individual capable of doing what needs to be done?** Although it's typical to give power of attorney to one's spouse, it's not wise to do so if your spouse can't balance a checkbook or isn't familiar with your business operations.

❑ **Is this individual readily available to go wherever you need?** It doesn't make sense to give power of attorney to someone who can't get to your bank, business or hospital bed when necessary.

Hard to Revoke?

Sometimes it's easier to grant a power of attorney than to revoke it. In some states, all you need to do is tell the person to give back the power-of-attorney document. However, if that person refuses or has skipped town, you will have to send a written document to all the parties that could be affected (such as banks, lenders, title companies, suppliers and creditors), stating that the power of attorney is canceled.

Furthermore, if the attorney in fact might be able to transact business in another locale (say, you live in Virginia and have a condo in Florida), you'll probably need to file a document revoking the power of attorney in that jurisdiction as well. The potential difficulty of canceling the power of attorney should make you extremely cautious in selecting who will serve as your attorney in fact.

❑ **Does this individual have the time to do it?** Performing the duties of an attorney in fact can consume a lot of hours for weeks, months or years—time that could interfere with the person's other responsibilities.

❑ **Is this person willing to be your attorney in fact?** Face it. Not everyone wants the added responsibility, particularly when it may require making controversial decisions, such as selling family heirlooms or authorizing risky surgery.

TYPES OF POWER OF ATTORNEY: STRONG AND WEAK

There are several types of power of attorney, each of which you can customize to fit your specific needs. If you have a lot of assets to protect, you should consult with an attorney who specializes in estate planning. Otherwise, all you may need is a book of legal forms, available at a stationery or office supply store or the public library. You will have to fill out the form in the presence of a notary public, but most banks (and hospitals) provide notary services free or for a nominal charge.

Caution: *If you go to a lawyer, ask upfront what the fee will be.* Some people have been charged as much as $2,000 for a regular power of attorney, which is typically just two pages long. Normally, a lawyer will charge $150 or less to prepare two copies of the document (one for you to give to your attorney in fact and another one—not a photocopy, but a second, notarized original—for you to keep in a safe place). The documents often can be prepared while you wait, and most firms have a notary on staff who will witness your signature at no extra charge.

A limited power of attorney

The so-called **regular power of attorney** is the kind you would use in the scenario where your neighbor agrees to collect your mail while you're away. A regular power of attorney specifies the responsibilities you are transferring to your named attorney in fact. Because she cannot do anything that is not spelled out in the document, it is also called a **limited power of attorney**.

There are several drawbacks to a limited power of attorney if you become incapacitated. First, your attorney in fact may not be able to do certain things for you because you didn't spell them out. For example, the document might not say that your attorney in fact can represent you in a lawsuit or collect money that you're owed. There's also the reverse problem: Your power-of-attorney document may be worded so vaguely or ambiguously that it could be interpreted as transferring powers you never intended. For instance, it might say the attorney in fact can "do, execute, and perform and finish for me and in my name all those things which shall be expedient and necessary." That's leaving a lot of wiggle room—including selling your business, revoking a trust or auctioning your rare stamp collection.

The most significant problem is that a limited power of attorney *ceases* when you become mentally incompetent—which is when the power of attorney is needed most. In this case, a judge will have to appoint a **guardian** (someone to take care of your health and welfare) and/or a **conservator** (someone to protect your assets) for however long you remain unconscious or mentally impaired.

Note: There are several reasons for trying to avoid the need for a conservatorship. First, the process of appointing a conservator takes place in open court, which could be embarrassing (there will be a public record of the fact that you are incapable of handling your own affairs) and, depending on your financial situation, harmful to your business. Second, you don't get to choose your guardian/conservator—the judge could appoint your least favorite relative, if that person is sufficiently persuasive. Third, your conservator will be required to file reports indicating how your assets are being managed, which is good protection for you but can be an overwhelming burden if that person is also your primary caregiver. Then there's the expense of hiring attorneys and calling in doctors to testify about your mental condition; the delay involved in going through the judicial system; and the equally time-consuming and expensive process of winding down the conservatorship when it's no longer needed.

Durable power of attorney

To prevent your transfer of authority from ending when you become incapacitated, you should grant a **durable power of attorney** to your attorney in fact. To avoid the problem of inadvertently omitting essential powers (such as being able to endorse checks in your name), it should also be a **general power of attorney**.

If you do not execute a durable power of attorney prior to becoming incapacitated, your affairs will hang in limbo until you are mentally competent to understand what you are signing and physically capable of making at least an *X* on the signature line. While this is for your protection, it can play havoc with your finances if you are seriously ill or injured yet are not so far gone that an incompetency proceeding should take place.

Observation: *Some physicians treat almost any sign of life as an indication of competency, while others are more discriminating. If you find yourself in the situation where you need a hospitalized family member to give you her power of attorney, you are well advised to wait until there is no doubt she understands what's going on. For one, the notary could decline to certify that the patient willingly and with full knowledge signed the document. But even if the notary certifies the document, another family member could allege that you coerced the patient into signing and could request that a judge void the power of attorney and hold you liable for everything you did while claiming to be the attorney in fact. In the case of my husband, it was two months after his stroke before we both felt comfortable with his giving me power of attorney, even though I'd had the document drawn up during the third week of his hospitalization.*

➤ **Recommendation:** *Execute a durable power of attorney now, while there's no question about your competency.*

Although the wording of a general power of attorney focuses on protecting your financial assets, it essentially gives your attorney in fact the power to make virtually any decision and transaction on your behalf. That's because almost everything you can imagine can have an impact on your assets, for better or worse—whether it be wallpapering your kitchen, returning library books or buying groceries. Just in case the wording doesn't stretch to cover a particular activity, the general power of attorney typically includes a clause saying, in essence, "This general power of attorney includes anything I forgot to mention."

If you're worried about giving your attorney in fact such broad control, another approach is to give a **durable limited power of attorney**, which spells out in excruciating detail exactly what your attorney in fact can do. For example, instead of saying that she can "sell real estate," the power of attorney would stipulate the type of property, legal description, address and so on, as well as the specific powers you are transferring, such as the ability to mortgage, sell or buy.

Be aware, however, that even a durable power of attorney can be problematic. Some institutions have little experience with this type of document and, therefore, are very cautious about accepting it at face value. For example, some banks and brokerages may require you to use their own forms; others require the durable power of attorney to be renewed (that is, signed by the grantor) at regular intervals, such as every five years. These can be insurmountable obstacles if you are incapacitated at the time, which would defeat the whole purpose of the durable power of attorney.

➤ **Recommendation:** *You can avoid some potential problems by asking your bank, brokerage or other financial institutions about any special requirements and complying with them. Alternatively, your lawyer could add a clause to your durable power of attorney stating that refusal to accept it will subject that institution to litigation.*

Once you've executed a durable power of attorney, you should give it to your attorney in fact right away to keep in a safe place, with the understanding that the power of attorney is not to be used unless, and until, you become incapacitated. Meanwhile, you continue to conduct business as usual. In reality, though, the power of attorney is *effective immediately*, meaning that your attorney in fact could transact business under your name at the same time you are handling your business affairs. Obviously, this can be problematic, particularly if your attorney in fact turns out to be a bad apple.

Springing durable power of attorney

One way to prevent this is to use a **springing durable power of attorney**, which is activated only when you become incompetent. Unfortunately, it requires that a judge declare you incompetent, which can give rise to problems similar to those related to a regular, or limited, power of attorney.

In many jurisdictions, the judge will hold incompetency hearings directly at the hospital, usually in a small, private meeting room. The judge's docket may even include regularly scheduled hours one or two days a month at the local hospital for that purpose. A potential difficulty may arise, however, if the doctors can't agree on your incompetency.

Caution: *Not all states recognize a springing power of attorney.* In that case, simply make your durable power of attorney **conditional** on two physicians' certification that you are not mentally competent. Similar language can be used for determining when your disability has passed.

➤ **Recommendation:** *If you're concerned about your attorney in fact exercising the durable power of attorney while you are healthy and able to conduct all your business affairs yourself, give the actual document to someone else, such as your lawyer, to give to your attorney in fact if and when you become incapacitated. More to the point, though, is that if you're concerned about your attorney in fact misusing your power of attorney, you should select another person for the task.*

GRANTING A MEDICAL POWER OF ATTORNEY

Because a durable general power of attorney covers virtually every aspect of your affairs, some lawyers say it is the only document you need if your assets are under about $625,000. But your state's laws and courts might say otherwise. For example, in many states, a durable general power of attorney does not grant authority to make health care decisions, although, arguably, such decisions can have the greatest impact on your financial affairs.

To be on the safe side, you should complete a **durable power of attorney for health care**, also known as a **durable medical power of attorney**. This document lets you appoint a person (or persons) to make health care decisions for you when you are unable to do so yourself.

Be aware that the durable medical power of attorney cannot typically be exercised unless two or more physicians certify that you are incompetent. However, a judicial determination of incompetency is normally not required.

Each state has its own rules regarding durable medical powers of attorney. Generally, once you've signed one, it remains valid for as long as you live. However, if you move to another state, the durable medical power of attorney might not be legally valid. A lawyer will be able to determine that for you. (Some states, like Virginia, provide the form for a durable medical power of attorney at no cost via the Internet, along with clearly written instructions for filling it out.)

Typically, the durable medical power of attorney authorizes your agent to:

- Consent to, refuse or withdraw consent to any type of medical care, including that which might hasten your death.
- Request, receive and review any medical information regarding your health.
- Employ and discharge your health care providers.
- Authorize your admission, discharge and transfer to or from any medical care facility.
- Take any lawful actions necessary to carry out the health care decisions, including requesting a court order that requires your medical providers to administer or withdraw specific medical care.

Note: The durable medical power of attorney is not limited to situations where your condition is terminal. Furthermore, you can list very specific instructions in the document, including which medicines you do or do not want and how long you wish to remain on life support.

Even in states that recognize the durable medical power of attorney, your physician might not be legally required to follow any instruction that he considers ethically or medically inappropriate. In that case, the law may require the physician to make a reasonable effort to transfer you to another doctor.

➤ **Recommendation:** *Discuss your durable medical power of attorney with your primary care physician*

Why You Need a Will

A durable general power of attorney cannot authorize your attorney in fact to execute a will or other testamentary instrument on your behalf. Why do you need a will? If you don't have a will when you die, all your assets will pass to your heirs according to the laws of the state in which you live (your **state of domicile**). In legal jargon, anyone who dies without a will dies **intestate**, and the state's intestacy laws take over.

Because state intestacy laws are designed to be "one size fits all," they are not likely to coincide with your own wishes for distributing your assets to your family. And, of course, intestacy laws are not meant to help you save on estate taxes. If you die without a will, your family's estate tax bill will be maximized, not minimized. Moreover, an estate that is subject to intestacy laws may incur additional administrative expenses. If you die intestate and a minor child is a beneficiary, the disposition of those assets will probably be subject to a court order.

Reminder: *Once you have drawn up a will, be sure to review it regularly and keep it up to date with your financial and health situations. Also, if you move to another state, you should have an attorney in your new state of residence review your will to ensure it conforms to the legal requirements of that jurisdiction.*

to be sure there are no obstacles to his performing your stated desires. It is also a good idea to notify your insurance company that you have signed a durable medical power of attorney and to provide the insurer with the name, address and phone number of the person you've designated as your health care agent.

LIVING WILL APPLIES TO TERMINAL CONDITION

In addition to or in place of a durable medical power of attorney, you may also want to sign an **advance medical directive**, also called a **living will**. Unlike the durable medical power of attorney, a living will applies only when your attending physician determines that you have a terminal condition. If you sign a living will, you need to provide a copy to your physician before it can be implemented. (Again, the physician might not be legally required to follow your instructions, but usually the law demands that some attempt be made to honor your wishes.)

The basic purpose of a living will is to express your legal right to refuse life-prolonging procedures and be permitted to die naturally. If you want only certain procedures (for example, CPR but not feeding tubes), you can specify that as well.

Some advisers say it's not necessary to have a living will in place because essentially all hospitals must now ask patients at the time of admission whether they have a living will and, if not, provide the form to patients who so desire. However, it is probably preferable to fill out a living will in advance, when you're not under stress.

Just as with a regular will, you should review your living will from time to time, especially if there is a change in your health or family status. If you decide to change your living will, simply fill out a new one and give a copy to your physician. Don't forget to retrieve and destroy all the earlier copies. You can also revoke your living will at any time, either by telling your physician or by giving him a written statement, depending on what your state law requires.

Note: States that recognize living wills typically provide that, if you die as a consequence of the directive's being followed, your death will not be considered a suicide for purposes of any life insurance you are carrying.

THE RIGHT WAY TO KEEP RECORDS

Let's assume you have selected someone to step into your shoes if you become medically disabled. The next issue to address is how you will convey important information to that person if you are unable to communicate or, as frequently happens in the case of serious illness or injury, simply cannot remember things.

For that matter, could you tell that person right now, off the top of your head, the name of your insurance company? Or where, in the pile of papers you've shoved in a drawer, is the booklet explaining your health insurance coverage? Do you remember whether you filled out and returned the form that lets you take money out of your mutual fund by phone? And where did you put that bank slip confirming the instructions you gave about your CD or Roth IRA?

Looking toward the future, have you ever indicated who should be your children's guardian if you're incapacitated? Have you told anyone that you've already purchased a burial plot? Does anyone know whom you would want to serve as your pallbearers?

Or, on a somewhat cheerier note, were you aware that the government will cancel your guaranteed student loan if you become permanently disabled? Did you know that you may be able to make certain penalty-free withdrawals from your IRA and 401(k) plans for medical emergencies? Have you checked to see whether your life insurance policy has a provision that lets you skip payments if you are disabled?

In short, there's a ton of information that needs to be conveyed to your "deputy" in an emergency. Some of that information is lying around your house; some is carried around in your head. Some of it may or may not be important, but your "second-in-command" would be able to find out—provided you leave enough clues for him or her to follow.

Laying out the clues

Accordingly, there are three steps you need to take in advance of a medical crisis:

1. Collect and sort all the important papers, keys, phone numbers and other tangibles that relate to your household and to your personal, business and financial affairs.

2. Write down all the combination numbers, code words, phone numbers and other key information that you have memorized.

3. Round up all the personal papers that prove who you are, how long you've been around and what you've been up to. These papers—and anything else that might indicate your eligibility for financial or social service benefits—may entail contacting the hospital where you were born, the court that issued your marriage certificate or divorce decree, your college alumni office and other institutions to get copies of records that you might not have.

Similarly, there are three places where you need to keep certain records:

1. A fireproof home safe ("firebox"), business firebox, locked file cabinet or bank safe deposit box: for records (including floppy disks) that are difficult to replace.

2. An easily accessible file cabinet in your home or business: for records that you frequently update or refer to.

3. A records "archive," which can be as simple as cardboard boxes in the attic or a closet: for older documents (such as tax records and insurance policies from previous years), which you might need as proof in an audit or a lawsuit.

Finally, you will need to create a master list, or "Answers Book," indicating what items you have and where you've put them. If you have a home computer, you can compile and keep your master list there. But you should also keep a current copy on a floppy disk as well as a hard-copy backup.

HOW TO COMPILE YOUR RECORDS

Your life has different facets—work, family, finances—each of which has its own requisite "instructions." The best way to begin organizing all these facets into neat, complete files is to focus on one aspect of your life at a time.

The approach described in this section is simply a method to get you started and help ensure that nothing crucially important is left out. When you actually start putting your documents, keys, instructions and so forth into their respective storage places, you should adopt a labeling system for your files that makes sense to you and, eventually, to your "second in command."

Here's an overview of the general categories you should consider as you go about compiling your records:

Family Matters

- Household "answers" (phone numbers, location of keys, etc.)
- Emergency consent forms for each child
- Trust-related information
- Birth and marriage certificates
- Divorce or separation papers
- Adoption papers
- Citizenship papers
- Military service documents
- Household special instructions (yard care, garbage pickup, etc.)
- Personal history (birthplace, mother's maiden name, etc.)
- Funeral and burial instructions
- Persons to notify in case of your death
- Will-related information
- Letter of instruction (besides your will)
- Living will

Finances

- Bank accounts
- Credit card accounts
- CDs
- Annuity policies and plans
- Profit-sharing plans
- Gold coins, art and antiques
- Other assets
- Income tax returns
- Accounts and notes receivable
- Installment purchases
- Personal financial statement
- Safe deposit box
- Stocks and bonds (broker's name, location of certificates, etc.)
- Retirement plans
- Stock option plans
- Limited partnerships
- Social Security number
- Personal loans
- Other loan agreements and information

Properties

- Real estate
- Autos, other motor vehicles, boats
- Receipts on major improvements
- License receipts

Insurance Policies

- Life
- Major medical
- Health
- Long-term care
- Disability
- Property
- Auto/boat
- Other insurance (equipment, credit card, hospital indemnity, etc.)

Business

- Business information (bank accounts, instructions for sale, etc.)
- Income and property records
- Canceled checks
- Receipts
- Contracts
- Tax records
- Insurance policies
- Partnership agreement
- Buy-sell agreement
- Joint-venture records

LIFE'S LITTLE INSTRUCTION BOOK

As you begin compiling documentation for the five categories outlined on page 53, you'll probably start thinking of numerous details that you carry around in your head or have scribbled on a memo pad beside the telephone or have stuck with magnets on the refrigerator door. Yes, you need to gather all that minutia and add it to your life's little instruction book. To help jog your memory, the following "nag lists" are as good as it gets:

Household Answers

- Fire department phone number ____________
- Police phone number ____________
- Home address, phone, fax, e-mail address, computer password(s) ____________
- Office address, phone number ____________
- Beeper number ____________
- Car phone number ____________
- Cellular phone number ____________
- Car make, model, color, license number ____________
- Neighbor's name, home phone, address, office phone ____________
- Another neighbor's name, home phone, address, office phone ____________
- Best friend's name, home phone, address, office phone ____________
- Closest relative's name, home phone, address, office phone ____________
- Location of extra house key, electrical breaker box, water cutoff, thermostat, alarm system box, etc. ____________
- List of all your medications, dosages and prescribing physician (available from your pharmacist) ____________

Name, phone number of:

- Your clergyman ____________
- Security alarm company ____________
- Doctor ____________
- Hospital ____________
- Local ambulance service ____________
- Dentist ____________
- Orthodontist ____________
- Eye doctor ____________
- Medical specialists ____________
- Pharmacy ____________
- Veterinarian ____________
- Electrician ____________
- Plumber ____________
- Air conditioning/heating company ____________
- Appliance repair company ____________

Household Special Instructions

Schedules and contacts for:

- Yard care ______
- Garbage pickup ______
- Newspapers ______
- Other subscriptions (expiration dates) ______
- Animals (instructions, kennels) ______
- Warranties, maintenance contracts (appliances, etc.) ______

Personal History

- Your full name (especially if you go by initials, middle name or nickname) and maiden name ______
- Your marital/domestic partner status ______
- Spouse's name, maiden name, date of birth, birthplace, Social Security number ______
- Previous spouse's name, maiden name, address, phone number, date of birth, Social Security number ______
- Current address (length of residence) ______
- Previous addresses (as far back as you can remember) ______
- Date of birth and birthplace (city, county, state or country) ______
- Father's name and mother's married/maiden names ______
- Your spouse's mother's maiden name (*believe it or not, the Social Security Administration, for one, may ask this question*) ______
- Your children's names, dates of birth, birthplaces, Social Security numbers (indicate natural, adopted or stepchildren) ______
- Your brothers' and sisters' names, phone numbers ______
- Major illness/surgery information (type of surgery, hospital or clinic name, dates of admission/discharge, attending physician) ______
- Military service: serial number, enlistment/discharge dates, current rank or rank at discharge ______
- Your occupation title and employment contacts (supervisor, personnel office, employee assistance hotline, etc.) ______

- Schools attended (name, location, degree, dates of attendance and graduation) ____________
- Church membership or affiliation ____________
- Fraternal, service, social, union and other memberships ____________
- Special recognitions and awards (*in fact, your current résumé would be handy)* ____________

Funeral and Burial Instructions

- Clergyman or other whom you'd like to have officiate (name, phone number) ____________
- Funeral home preference ____________
- Location of service (church, graveside, etc.) ____________
- Cemetery plot or mausoleum slot purchased (name of cemetery, address; lot number; copy of deed) ____________
- Prepaid funeral plan number ____________
- Viewing wishes (open or closed casket) ____________
- Special requests for funeral service and burial (casket or cremation; music selections; biblical passages; type of clothing, etc.) ____________
- Your preference for charitable donations if in lieu of flowers ____________
- Organ donor certification (on driver's license or a witnessed form) ____________

Will Information

- Location of original will and date ____________
- Attorney's name, address, phone number ____________
- Executor's name, address, phone number ____________

Trust Information

- Name of trust ____________
- Location of original trust document ____________
- Date of trust ____________
- Attorney's name, address, phone number ____________
- Trustee's name, address, phone number ____________

Advisers

Name, phone number, address of:

- Clergy ____________
- Attorney ____________
- Banker ____________
- Accountant ____________
- Stock broker ____________
- Financial adviser ____________
- Insurance agent ____________
- Realtor ____________
- Other advisers ____________

Bank Accounts

- Account names, numbers____________________
- Bank name, address, phone number of branch you use ____________________
- Type of account (joint, individual, checking, savings, etc.) ____________________
- Person(s) authorized to sign ____________________
- Bank officer to contact (name, phone number)____________________
- Where you keep checkbook/savings passbook ____________________
- Special benefits (overdraft protection, life insurance, etc.)____________________
- CD maturity date; any special instructions____________________
- IRA account information____________________

Safe Deposit Box

- Bank name, address, phone number ____________________
- Location of keys (two keys are given for each box) ____________________
- Persons authorized to sign* ____________________
- Contents ____________________

*Consider authorizing a friend, as well as your spouse, to sign in case of emergency. You don't have to give them a key to the safe deposit box; just tell them where you keep it.

Credit Cards

- Card issuer's name, phone number, billing address ____________________
- Card number ____________________
- Where you usually keep the card ____________________
- Person(s) authorized to sign ____________________
- Special features** ____________________

**Accidental death and dismemberment insurance when you charge airline or train tickets, "good customer" free life insurance policy, reduced car rental rates, insurance covering your monthly minimum payment if you're disabled, etc.

Stocks and Bonds

- Brokerage firm's name, address____________________
- Broker's name, phone number ____________________
- Account name(s), number(s) ____________________
- Stock you hold individually: name of company; number of shares; location of certificate(s) ____________________
- Savings Bonds: date(s) of maturity; redemption value; name, phone number of any co-owner ____________________

Other Assets

- Type of asset (retirement plan, annuity contract, stock option plan, etc.) and where the information is kept ____________________
- Appraisals (and photographs) of antiques, art or other valuables ____________________
- Receipts of purchase, repairs, etc.____________________

- If a tangible asset, where it's located______________________________
- Any instructions from you about liquidating, distributing or contributing the asset ____

Retirement Plan(s)

- Name of fund______________________________
- Institution administering fund (name, address, phone number)____
- Amount in fund (as of today's date) ________________________
- Date funds (or a portion) are retrievable________________________
- Name of person(s) funds are available to ________________________
- Additional information (beneficiary, phone number and your PIN number for accessing the account) ________________________

Loan Information

- Amount and date of loan ________________________
- Loan number ________________________
- Lender's name, address, phone number________________________
- Collateral (what and where it is) ________________________
- Interest rate________________________
- Number and amount of payments ________________________
- Due date, late date, final payment date ________________________
- Location of loan agreement ________________________
- Reason for loan ________________________
- Additional information (such as an insurance policy that would cover the monthly payments if you became disabled)________________________

Accounts and Notes Receivable

- Debtor's name, address, home and business phone number ____
- Date and amount of loan ________________________
- Terms of payment ________________________
- Location of agreement ________________________
- Additional information (such as name, address, phone number of collection agency you use) ________________________

Real Estate

- Property address, description________________________
- Owners' names, addresses, phone numbers ________________________
- Date of purchase, purchase price ________________________
- Name, address, phone number of mortgagor ________________________
- Approximate mortgage balance as of today's date ________________________
- Number of years on mortgage________________________
- Interest rate________________________
- Loan number ________________________
- Payment amount ________________________

- Due date, late date, final payment date ____________
- Property taxes and due date ____________
- Location of title/deed ____________
- Description, date, cost of major improvements ____________
- Location of receipts ____________

Auto or Other Motor Vehicles

- Make, model, year, ID number ____________
- License number ____________
- Registered owner(s) ____________
- Date purchased ____________
- Seller's name, address, phone number ____________
- Name, address, phone number of lender ____________
- Title number, location of title ____________
- Safety/emissions inspections dates ____________
- Maintenance information ____________
- Family licensed drivers (names, license numbers; if out-of-state license, indicate state) ____________

Life Insurance

- Name of insured ____________
- Amount and date issued ____________
- Maturity date ____________
- Cash value as of today's date ____________
- Beneficiary ____________
- Owner of policy ____________
- Insurance company's name, address, phone number ____________
- Agent's name, phone and fax numbers ____________
- Policy number ____________
- Premium amount and due dates ____________
- How premium is paid (bank draft, check, salary allotment, etc.) ____________
- Location of policy ____________
- Details (such as any provision to pay premiums if you're disabled) ____________

Health and Other Insurance

- Named individual(s) covered by policy ____________
- Insurance company's name, address, phone number ____________
- Agent's name, phone, fax number ____________
- Policy number ____________
- Deductible (annual and lifetime) ____________
- Premium amount and due dates ____________
- How premium is paid (bank draft, check, salary allotment, etc.) ____________
- Location of policy ____________
- Details of coverage and exclusions ____________

What Goes Where

As you're pulling together all your records, you might as well start putting them in their proper places. This step may also help you identify items that you need to make additional copies of, want to amend or have to replace.

What to keep in a fire-proof box

What should you keep in a firebox? Things that you might need immediately or hard-to-replace items that you might not be able to retrieve right away from a bank safe deposit box. These include the following:

- Your will and your living will
- Your power of attorney (unless you've already given it to your attorney in fact)
- Life insurance policies and backup materials
- Birth certificate, passport and marriage certificate
- All documents relating to a separation or divorce
- Military service records (especially DD-214s)
- Citizenship or adoption papers
- Diplomas and licenses
- Permits (for example, a zoning permit for your home business)
- Union cards (unless you carry them with you)
- Social Security card (unless you carry this with you)
- Health records (particularly dates of vaccinations, operations)
- Receipts for high-cost purchases (furs, antiques, etc.)
- Receipts and canceled checks for home improvements
- Records of purchase, property descriptions, proofs of ownership and insurance (deeds, titles, surveys, etc.)
- Receipts for paid-off debts
- Records of money owed to you
- Employment contracts

(You can buy a firebox with a UL 350-degree half-hour rating for about $30 from an office supply store.)

What to keep in a safe deposit box

- Current homeowner's, tenant's and auto insurance policies
- Appraisals/sales slips for valuables
- Household inventory, including any photos and sales receipts
- List of numbers and locations of all retirement accounts (Keogh plans, IRAs, etc.)
- Stocks and other securities
- Bonds and Treasury securities
- List of U.S. Savings Bonds (denominations, serial numbers, issue dates)

- Gold coins and other precious metals
- Original prospectus and sales material for any limited partnerships
- Names, account numbers of mutual funds and unit trusts
- Trust documents

What to keep in a filing cabinet

Everything else should go in your filing cabinet (records that are current or no older than three years or so) or a records archive. Documents that you should keep in a filing cabinet include these:

- Health, disability and long-term-care insurance policies
- Tax records
- Bank records
- Paycheck stubs
- Receipts for paid bills
- Medical and drug bills
- Monthly credit card statements
- Mortgage, bank loan, installment purchase contracts and other debts
- Annual statements about pension, profit-sharing, salary-deferral or employee thrift plan
- Retirement plan documents, along with annual reports
- Brokerage house agreements, annual statements, dividend reinvestment statements, confirmations of trades; any related correspondence or telephone notes
- Rental property income and expense records
- Home business income and expense records
- Receipts for tax-deductible gifts
- Your cemetery deed, material for your obituary, funeral instructions and a copy of your living will

YOUR BOOK OF ANSWERS

You're almost done! All that's left to do is record the results of your data collection on a master list or "Answers Book." Be sure to tell the person you've designated as your "deputy" where to find it. For example, give the person the file name if it's on your computer or the combination if it's locked in your home safe, or you might even just make her a copy of the list. Now you are prepared for almost any disaster. . . .

Part II

Maintaining Cash Flow in a Medical Crisis

Your financial health during a medical crisis will depend to a great extent on how well you've prepared your safety net. At a minimum, that will require (1) emergency funds for at least 90 days, (2) health insurance and (3) a durable general power of attorney.

Ideally, you will also have the following:

- Disability insurance if you're employed.
- A medical power of attorney.
- An "Answers Book" of instructions for your attorney in fact.
- Long-term-care insurance.
- Life insurance.
- A living will.
- A master list of all your assets.
- A will.

But if a medical catastrophe strikes before your safety net is in place, you might still be able to land on your feet by taking advantage of government, medical and other assistance. Therefore, in addition to giving you an opportunity to review your preparations before they're put to the test, Part II offers some guidance about backup measures that may help you over certain rough spots.

Life Is What Happens While You're Busy Making Plans 4

Earlier this week, one of our friends was diagnosed with cancer. He is self-employed, supports his wife and mother and has no health insurance. In five months he will be 65 years old and eligible for Medicare. To help defray his expenses, his friends are raffling off a TV set, selling chances at $10 each.

Obviously, raffling off a TV isn't going to solve this man's problems, but there are ways you can forestall the same thing happening to you. Naturally, the best way to limit your medical-related financial risk is by staying healthy and avoiding undue physical risks. You know the drill: Eat right, drink less, quit smoking, lose weight, exercise, get enough sleep, wear your seatbelt and so on.

The next best thing is to get early diagnosis and treatment of a medical problem. Many serious illnesses can be cured relatively inexpensively if they are nipped in the bud. Learn the warning signs for cancer, diabetes and other serious conditions. If you suspect you have a medical problem, don't ignore it with the hope that it will go away—it might only get worse. See a doctor immediately.

An Ounce of Prevention

You should get a complete physical at least every two to five years (annually, if you are age 40 or older). If you have health insurance, your checkup may cost as little as $5. Without insurance, the "regular and customary" charge where you live may be as high as $190 to $275, including an electrocardiogram. Remember: You may be able to deduct the cost of your physical exam and any related expenses (including the cost of transportation to and from the doctor's office) on Schedule A of your federal income tax return.

Observation: *Community health centers and other public health facilities generally provide free or low-cost routine physicals; screening and diagnostic tests for vision, hearing and other medical problems; and vaccinations for influenza and other diseases. To find out about a public health center in your community, call your local consumer affairs office (check your phone directory) or call the information line for federally qualified health centers (FQHC) at (800) 638-6833.*

If You're Diagnosed With a Serious Illness

Even though you may suspect you have a serious medical condition, the diagnosis confirming your fears is likely to come as a shock. What your doctor tells you about your

Tips on Choosing a Doctor

If you belong to a managed care plan, your choice of primary care physicians will be limited to "plan" or "preferred" doctors. Your plan will provide a list of physicians at the time you enroll. Before choosing a doctor, try to get recommendations from other doctors or nurses or from co-workers who consulted doctors in your managed care plan.

If your choice of physicians is not limited by your insurance plan, the best starting point is to ask doctors you know, friends, family and co-workers for their recommendations. You can also contact hospitals and doctor-referral services in your area.

Once you have the names of several doctors, call to make sure they're accepting new patients. You may also want to set up a "get acquainted" appointment with the physician. Be sure to ask what, if any, charge there will be for the visit.

Other sources of information about physicians include:

❑ ***The Directory of Medical Specialists,*** which contains information about some 400,000 practicing physicians and can be found in most public libraries.

❑ **"AMA Physician Select,"** which is the American Medical Association's free service on the Internet for information about physicians (http://www.ama-assn.org).

❑ **The American Board of Medical Specialties,** at (800) 776-2378, which can tell you whether a physician is board certified in a particular specialty.

❑ **Your state medical licensing board** (check the Blue Pages of your phone book), which can tell you if any complaints or disciplinary actions have been taken against a specific doctor.

disease and the possible treatments may get lost in the confusion of trying to come to grips with the reality of your illness.

As soon as you can, start learning as much about your medical condition as possible. This is important for several reasons:

- **Fear of the unknown may prevent you** from taking the actions necessary to improve your condition.
- **Knowledge of available treatments can be valuable** in dealing with your insurance company.
- **Understanding how your condition will affect your lifestyle** will help you determine whether you can work and what accommodations, if any, your employer will need to provide for you.

Find out what your insurance covers

If you're covered by an individual or group health insurance plan, you need to find out exactly what your insurer will pay for. Some plans exclude certain illnesses, such as Alzheimer's disease. Many plans cover only standard types of treatment and won't pay for experimental therapies used in treating AIDS, cancer and other diseases.

Plans vary widely on the amount you must pay before coverage starts. They also pay different percentages of the cost of various services. Some plans pay for only 30 days in the hospital; others cover many more. Some cover certain home care services; others don't. The number of days of rehabilitation covered will also vary. Remember, too, that most plans have limits on what they will pay toward treatment for a given health problem on an annual or lifetime basis. Most also have a ceiling on the total benefits you can receive.

Dealing With the Diagnosis

Upon hearing that you are seriously ill, you are likely to experience a host of emotions, ranging from initial denial to bottomless grief. These are common reactions. Try to understand the emotions you are feeling and use them to help you cope with the changes in your lifestyle and how they will affect your financial situation. Those emotions include:

- ✔ **Concern:** Although the diagnosis usually is definite once the test results have been examined, you may be concerned about its accuracy and the desirability of the recommended treatment. A second opinion from another source can be helpful and is often recommended. However, once the diagnosis and treatment have been agreed upon by two physicians, seeking a third opinion is unlikely to result in a more acceptable diagnosis—and probably would be a waste of money.
- ✔ **Fear:** Concern can quickly turn into fear about how the illness will progress, how successful the treatment will be, how the illness will impact your life and a whole lot of other unknowns. Because you may need to make many important decisions at this time—many of which may hinge on your insurance coverage—don't hesitate to ask your doctor for further explanations about your condition.
- ✔ **Denial:** This can be a helpful coping mechanism. However, you could make your condition worse—and more expensive to treat—if you convince yourself that nothing really is wrong.
- ✔ **Relief:** When you're given a definite diagnosis, you may feel a sense of relief because now you know what you're facing. Remember, though, that diagnosis is only a precursor to a cure. This is not the time to fold up your safety net, but rather the time to patch any holes in it.
- ✔ **Frustration:** If you suffer from a chronic or progressively debilitating disease, you are likely to feel frustrated as your illness increasingly affects your daily activities. Your insurance might cover devices such as canes, walkers and wheelchairs, or you may be able to obtain free or low-cost medical equipment through your local social services department or a charitable organization.
- ✔ **Unfairness:** Sometimes regarded as the "Why me?" syndrome, the feeling of being singled out or shortchanged is not uncommon. However, some 21 million Americans are living with chronic illness—you are not alone. Organizations such as the National Cancer Institute, (800) 4-CANCER, can provide information and support services that may help you feel less isolated.
- ✔ **Anger:** The inconveniences caused by your illness, the attitude of doctors and health care personnel, the lack of understanding from family and friends can lead to anger. By using your anger constructively, you may be able to change people's attitudes and get the help you need.
- ✔ **Loss of Control:** At some point, your disease becomes the determining factor in many situations. You might not be able to drive a car anymore, work or even dress yourself. By preparing for these eventualities, you can exert a certain amount of control over what happens to you and your affairs.
- ✔ **Devastation:** Financial loss, career loss and family disruption are the major sources of feelings of devastation. Again, you can do a lot to mitigate these problems by preparing your safety net as best you can. And here's a heretical thought: Would it really be so terrible if you had to live on a smaller income, take a different job or change your household responsibilities?
- ✔ **Mourning:** The loss of your dreams and the person you once were must be permitted a period of mourning. You'll need to readjust your expectations to fit the new reality. Look to your local social services agency or department of vocational and rehabilitative services for help in setting new goals.
- ✔ **Humbling:** You're likely to experience a change in perspective and attitude as you realize how many aspects of life depend on one's health. Indeed, your health suddenly seems much more important than your financial security. Just remember, though, money is what pays for your health care.
- ✔ **Acceptance:** With education, support and time, you can learn to accept your medical condition and concentrate on treatment. You may still hope for a possible cure, but you know better than to waste your money in search of a "medical miracle."

Caution: *Many plans require precertification or preauthorization for hospitalization and treatment.* If you are covered by a group health plan, you might have all the preapprovals lined up for your treatment—when suddenly your employer changes health plans. This will send you back to square one. If the new insurer refuses to approve your treatment, ask your employer to contact the insurer. In this case your employer, rather than your doctor, may be in the best position to negotiate coverage with the new insurance company.

➤ **Recommendation:** *Read your insurance coverage carefully and, if possible, clear up gray areas before you incur a lot of expenses. If you have a group plan, it's often best to have your doctor or a hospital financial representative deal with the insurance company—the medical professionals generally know the right buzzwords to use and can be helpful in advocating coverage on your behalf. If you have an individual plan, your insurance agent may be able to get quick answers to your questions, saving you time and worry.*

Also, keep in mind that misdiagnoses happen frequently in emergency rooms. This can lead to the denial of claims that later turn out to be valid. If you find the need to dispute a denied claim, your insurance agent, Employee Assistance Program personnel or hospital financial representative should be able to help you. Be sure to save all the paperwork you receive from the hospital.

Be an active partner in your treatment

Developing a partnership with your doctor is extremely important. In particular, you should discuss any personal circumstances that will affect your treatment. These issues include the following:

- If you are insured, whether your insurance will cover your treatment.
- If you are not insured, whether you will need financial assistance.
- Whether you have family or friends who can provide transportation to the doctor's office or health care facility.
- If you live alone and will need help taking your medication, eating, bathing, etc.
- Whether you will need devices to assist you in getting around in your home, car or office.

Keeping an open line of communication with your doctor can help you gain control over your illness, its prognosis and any treatment options. Ask questions, and take notes or tape-record your meetings with the doctor. It's also a good idea to have your spouse or another family member sit in on your consultations. That person's questions can help clarify information provided by the doctors. Also, being aware of your illness, prognosis and possible treatment will help that family member better handle the role of being your health care advocate, if that becomes necessary later.

Don't Be Suckered by 'Miracle Cures'

Americans waste billions of dollars on useless remedies and health-related devices that are advertised in magazines, on TV and elsewhere, according to the Federal Trade Commission. Chasing after a miracle cure not only can ruin you financially but also may seriously compromise your health by delaying appropriate treatment.

Recognize the typical phrases used to tout worthless products. The FTC recommends watching out for these "tricks of the trade":

- Does the ad promise a "quick and easy cure"?
- Is the product advertised as effective for a wide range of ailments or for an undiagnosed pain?
- Does the promoter use words such as "miraculous," "exclusive," "secret" or "ancient"?
- Is the product advertised as available from only one source, requiring payment in advance?
- Does the promoter use undocumented case histories that sound too good to be true?

Protect your resources from costly 'medical heroics'

Now is the time to pay close attention to protecting your financial resources from being depleted in a fruitless effort to perform a medical miracle. If you still haven't signed a durable power of attorney for health care and a living will (*see Section 3*), this might be your last opportunity to do so.

If you've already signed a durable medical power of attorney and a living will, make sure these documents continue to reflect your wishes. Having an actual diagnosis (and possibly, prognosis) of your medical condition gives you a valuable opportunity to address specific issues that could arise during your treatment.

IF YOU HAVE A DREAD DISEASE AND ARE UNINSURED . . .

Once you've been diagnosed with a severe medical problem, most commercial insurers won't sell you a policy. Don't even think about lying on your application either. You're likely to get caught when the insurance company checks your medical background when you file your application or submit a claim.

If you're no longer healthy, here are some options you might want to consider for obtaining coverage:

❑ **Call several large insurance plans in your region**, such as Blue Cross/Blue Shield or an HMO that advertises locally, and ask about their open enrollment periods. "Open enrollment" means that everyone who applies—AIDS patients included—is accepted at standard rates. Be aware, however, that under the Health Insurance Portability and Accountability Act of 1996 (HIPAA), insurers that market group health plans are allowed to impose exclusions for pre-existing conditions on new enrollees for up to 12 months. Therefore, if your medical condition is immediately life-threatening or you expect to undergo expensive treatment within the next 12 months, this probably is not a good option.

The Medical Information Bureau

The Medical Information Bureau is a repository of medical and certain nonmedical information about some 12 million Americans who have applied for insurance. The MIB was set up essentially to catch insurance cheats by serving as a clearinghouse for information obtained by insurers about applicants and policyholders. About 700 insurance companies are members of MIB. They must inform you in writing that your health information may be reported to MIB and receive your written authorization before sharing such information with other member insurers.

Medical information that MIB collects includes:

- Specific illnesses
- Suicide attempts
- Overweight and underweight
- Drug addiction or alcoholism if confirmed by applicant or a medical source
- Pertinent X-rays and lab tests
- Occupational poisoning
- Family history of diseases
- Anything else an insurer considers medically suspicious, such as an odd squiggle on your electrocardiogram

Nonmedical information that MIB collects includes:

- Reckless driving records
- Amateur flying
- Hazardous sports
- Applications for more life insurance than seems warranted

You can obtain a free copy of your nonmedical file from the Medical Information Bureau at P.O. Box 105, Essex Station, Boston, MA 02112; phone (617) 426-3660. Upon your request, MIB will send your medical file to any medical professional you designate (doctor, nurse, dentist, pharmacist, etc.), who is expected to discuss it with you. You are entitled to correct or elaborate on any information in the record.

Note: By Jan. 1, 1999, large health plans will be required, under the Health Insurance Portability and Accountability Act of 1996, to begin submitting personal medical histories and financial data about all their policyholders to a central health information database. Small health plans will have until Jan. 1, 2000, to begin complying with the requirement.

❑ **If you are able to work and are willing to apply** for a job with a large company, you can get coverage under the employer's group health plan, usually without submitting a medical questionnaire. When the time comes that you can no longer work, you can keep this insurance at your own expense for up to 18 months (29 months if you're disabled). At the end of the 18 months, any health insurer that markets individual policies in your state is required, under HIPAA, to accept your application for individual coverage. Best of all, the insurance company can't impose a new pre-existing condition exclusion on your coverage, as long as you haven't let your coverage lapse for more than 62 days.

❑ **Similarly, your spouse might try for a job** at a company with a good group health policy. Many large plans don't require dependents to submit a medical questionnaire to receive their coverage.

If your spouse is currently under a group health plan under which she originally turned down dependent coverage, you might still be able to get coverage as a dependent if her plan offers subsequent "open enrollment" periods. Under the provisions of HIPAA, the only other way to get dependent coverage after having turned it down is if you had other coverage at the time of the original offering. In that case, the insurance plan is required to accept your application for dependent coverage during a "special enrollment" period held specifically for that purpose.

❑ **Ask an independent insurance agent** to try to locate an insurer that would be willing to insure you for a higher than normal premium. The extra expense (including the agent's commission) would be worth it because you'd have a policy that covers your particular medical condition.

❑ **Consider TV-advertised or mail-order policies** if you cannot qualify for any other coverage. Ordinarily, these plans are a waste of money because of long waiting periods for pre-existing conditions and low payments for covered illnesses or hospitalizations. If, however, the benefits are reasonable and you're entitled to payments from the first day of hospitalization, you might be able to defray enough of your expenses to keep yourself financially afloat.

Observation: *Some indemnity plans offered through credit card issuers are fairly reasonable. For a monthly premium of about $15 you may be able to buy a policy that pays $300 a day for a hospital stay. When considering such plans, however, be sure to note whether they cover only accidents, not illnesses, and if the payments continue for only a limited time.*

❑ **Find out if your state has a health insurance pool** for the uninsured (or uninsurable). Even before HIPAA, about half the states offered catastrophic care policies, usually with higher than normal premiums and high deductibles. Now, since the new law, states are encouraged, but not required, to offer alternative health insurance at affordable rates.

If you still can't get insurance

You've got a few options left, but most of them will require that you deplete your resources before qualifying. Moreover, the quality of health care you receive may not be as good as it would be under an insurance plan. Also, you may have to use a health care facility that is 100 miles or so from where you live. Some of those last-ditch options include:

❑ **If you served in the military**, contact the Department of Veterans Affairs to find out if you're eligible to use a government health care facility. Your dependents also might be eligible for some government health benefits.

❑ **Some voluntary health organizations** and other charitable organizations provide small sums to assist with medical treatment. Among these are the Leukemia Society of America and Cancer Care, Inc. in the New York/New Jersey/Connecticut area. You might also try your church, union or fraternal organization.

❑ **If you're willing to participate** in a research study that involves your medical condition, the medical treatment is usually free.

❑ **If you're not working**, unable to work or can work only a few hours per week, you may qualify for state assistance (welfare), including state and local hospitalization.

❑ **If your monthly income** is less than $500, you may be eligible for Social Security's Supplemental Security Income (SSI), which normally qualifies you for Medicaid. If you're not eligible for SSI, you may still qualify to receive Medicaid under the "Medically Needy" category. (*See Section 1.*)

❑ **If your income and assets** exceed the "Medically Needy" guidelines, you may be able to get a portion of your medical expenses paid through Medicaid once you've paid a certain amount yourself. Contact your local Social Security office for information.

❑ **If you are already receiving** Social Security retirement benefits and are on Medicare, you may be eligible for assistance in paying for your Medicare premiums and your deductibles. Contact your local Social Security office.

Decide How to Pay Your Expenses

At the first sign of a crisis, you need to look at your monthly budget and immediately eliminate or postpone any expenditures that needlessly drain your financial assets. This will help you maintain cash flow if you become unable to work. Cutting back on optional expenses will also leave you more money for any increased expenses arising out of your medical crisis—for example, higher phone bills because of long-distance calls to relatives and insurance companies.

If you never got around to writing down your budget but simply pay your bills as they arrive, you'll need to find whatever records you can—checkbook entries, receipts, etc.—and try to get a sense of what your typical monthly expenses are. Then you can set priorities, making sure that rent or mortgage payments, insurance premiums, telephone and utility bills, property taxes and the like are at the top of the list.

Make contingency plans

You'll want to make sure that nothing messes up your cash flow in the event that you yourself are unable to make deposits to your bank account or write checks to pay the bills. Probably the most efficient way is by giving a durable general power of attorney to someone who is financially reliable. *(See details in Section 3.)* If you have concerns about the person who will be your attorney in fact, consider giving that individual only a limited power of attorney or a springing power of attorney.

Also, remember that nothing beats direct deposit of paychecks and other income. It not only prevents the loss or theft of your checks but also gives you almost immediate access to the money even when you can't go to the bank. If your employer offers this option and you haven't taken advantage of it, sign up now. It may take anywhere from 10 days to six weeks to get it activated, so the sooner you act, the better.

➤ **Recommendation:** *Find out which of your regular creditors, such as the phone company, utility company and mortgage bank, accept electronic payment. Some 95 percent of the nation's banks can do an Electronic Funds Transfer (EFT)—your bank may call it Account Mover or Direct Debit—to pay certain bills automatically out of the money in your checking or savings account. Sign up for this service, and eliminate the worry of how your bills will be paid if you're hospitalized.*

If your bank operates several branches in your area, it's also a good idea to fill out a signature card at more than one branch. You may be surprised to learn that your bank has a branch near your local hospital—which could come in handy.

Don't leave your dependents high and dry

Many married couples have jointly owned bank accounts. This means that you both hold the money in the accounts and can access it individually. Make sure that your jointly owned accounts give each owner the **right of survivorship**. This should be specified on the bank document. Otherwise, it might be argued that you hold the accounts only as **tenants in common**. Under a tenant-in-common ownership, when one of the owners dies, that person's share (which doesn't necessarily have to be 50 percent) is distributed according to that person's will or, if that person dies without a will (intestate), according to the state's laws. Until the decedent's share is distributed, the account is frozen.

See whether any of your other assets—particularly those that can be easily converted into cash—should be jointly owned. These assets could include securities and other investments or real estate.

Caution: *Some states are "community property" states, which hold that most property acquired by either spouse during the marriage is owned by both, regardless of whose name is on it.* Unlike jointly owned property, community property usually goes through probate when one of the spouses dies. If you live in a community property state or have recently moved from one, you should seek legal advice about your financial affairs.

If you have a safe deposit box, find out whether the bank will freeze it, too, in the event of your death. If you are married, it's probably a good idea for you and your spouse to have separate safe deposit boxes. (That way, you can keep your important papers in your spouse's box and vice versa, thus avoiding the problem of being unable to retrieve the papers if the box is frozen.) Typically, a box rents for about $60 a year.

Remember that you may need immediate access to certain papers, including your living will and durable power of attorney. Keep these in a firebox at home or in your office. (*See Section 3 for which records to keep in your firebox.*)

Train someone to take up the slack

Until my husband was transferred to a hospital that I could get to by bus, I spent approximately $1,400 on taxi fares going to and from the hospital. Such was the price of my never having bothered to learn to drive a stick-shift, which is the only type of car we've ever owned.

Actually, the price was even greater because then I had to pay a driving school about $350 to teach me how to work the clutch and gearshift. And it cost us another $700 or so in cab fare until I finally worked up the nerve to drive my husband to his medical appointments. In other words, my failure to learn necessary driving skills prior to John's stroke meant the extra expenditure of nearly $2,500 in cash—at the very time when it was critical to cut down on extraneous expenses.

Failure to train someone to do the things you've been accustomed to doing can result in a significant drain on your emergency funds. Most of us know someone, usually elderly, who cannot drive a car or prepare a meal and has to depend on community services, such as special transportation vans or Meals-on-Wheels. However, there rarely is any public assistance for those who are neither needy nor elderly.

Then, too, some two-income families divide up budget responsibilities and do not necessarily keep tabs on each other's payment schedule. They may maintain two checking accounts, have different methods of depositing paychecks and even different styles of paying bills—one using a home computer to pay bills electronically, the other mailing checks or even paying bills in person. If one of you becomes ill, the other spouse (or whoever is the attorney in fact) needs to be able to take over basic banking and bill-paying responsibilities. This may involve temporarily consolidating existing funds into one bank account. It may also mean learning new skills, such as balancing a checkbook, or using electronic banking services, such as CheckFree, or authorizing automated deposits or payments.

Protections Under the ADA, FMLA

Two federal laws give you certain protections that may help you keep your job, even as your illness progresses. These laws are the Americans With Disabilities Act (ADA) and the Family and Medical Leave Act (FMLA). Because neither law applies to all employers, you should check with your employer's human resources manager about whether your state laws give you additional protections.

Under the ADA, employers with 15 or more employees are prohibited from discriminating against "qualified individuals with disabilities." You are considered to have a disability if you have a physical or mental impairment that substantially limits one or more major life activities, or have a record of such an impairment or are regarded as having such an impairment. The ADA prohibits discrimination in all employment practices, including job application procedures, hiring, firing, advancement, compensation, training and other employment-related activities. As long as your illness does not interfere with your ability to perform the "essential functions" of your job, your employer cannot fire you, demote you or force you to retire.

Because the law focuses on the "essential functions" of your job, you are protected even if you can't do some of the marginal functions of your job. If your disability does interfere with your ability to perform the essential functions of your job but you could still perform these duties if "reasonable accommodations" were made, your employer is required to provide those accommodations. Keep in mind, though, that a "reasonable accommodation" does not include reassigning an essential function of your job to another employee.

The FMLA enables eligible employees to take up to 12 weeks of unpaid, job-protected leave each year for the employee's own serious health condition, caring for a spouse or immediate family member with a serious health condition, or the birth/adoption/foster care of a child.

The law applies to all public agencies and to companies having 50 or more employees working within a 75-mile radius of the work site. About 40 percent of U.S. workers are covered by the law. Eligible employees must work for a covered employer for at least 12 months and clock at least 1,250 hours during the 12 months leading up to FMLA leave. If you are eligible for FMLA benefits, your employer is required to maintain your health insurance coverage as well as life insurance and disability benefits. In addition, the use of FMLA leave cannot result in the loss of any employment benefit that accrued prior to the start of your leave.

Your employer is allowed to require you to submit certification by your physician or other health care practitioner attesting to the fact that you are seriously ill. Typically, the certification asks for a diagnosis, probable duration of your condition and the prescribed treatment plan.

Observation: *Not many eligible employees are taking FMLA unpaid leave. Less than 2 percent of eligible employees used FMLA leave in 1996 among companies responding to the 1997 Employee Benefits Survey, conducted by the National Institute of Business Management, and the average amount of FMLA time they took was 5.5 weeks. Currently, Congress is considering proposals that would broaden the FMLA to include employers with 25 or more employees, which would extend the coverage to an estimated 14 percent more of the private work force.*

Making Ends Meet While You're a Patient

5

The hospital where the ambulance took my husband misdiagnosed his stroke symptoms as delirium tremens. In fact, he had five blood clots—one near his brain stem, which was causing convulsions. The doctors had to wait seven days for the convulsions to stop before they could run diagnostic tests. I knew that a misdiagnosis could mess up John's employment (involving a security clearance) as well as his insurance, disability income and long-term-care benefits. Fortunately, John's employer advanced him some sick leave until I could find out what his medical condition really was and activate his disability income and long-term-care insurance.

So began my odyssey through the world of filling out forms. My insurance agent faxed me the disability income and long-term-care claim forms, and John's co-workers brought me his employer's forms (two to justify the sick leave, another to put John on leave-without-pay status and a fourth to apply for his employer's leave-share program).

By this time, four weeks had passed, and John was in a third hospital, which meant he had a new "treating physician." This doctor could sign only the parts of the forms that dealt with John's prognosis; I had to go back to the previous doctor to sign the parts dealing with John's diagnosis. I showed up at that doctor's office—only to have a thunderstorm instantly knock out all the power. Undeterred, I dug a small flashlight out of my bag, turned it on and insisted that the doctor sign the forms then and there.

When You Land in the Hospital . . .

There are two ways to enter a hospital: feet first (that is, you come in and register yourself) or head first (on a stretcher, with someone else signing you in). The way you go in can definitely make a difference in what you pay out.

Walk-in registration

When you voluntarily enter a hospital, you have a certain amount of control over your expenses, particularly if you have time to plan ahead. If you have insurance, your policy probably requires you or your doctor to get preapproval to use a particular hospital. This ensures that you pay the least amount out of pocket. If you will be undergoing elective surgery, your insurance plan may also require you to get a second opinion before providing coverage.

Caution: *If you're insured through an HMO or other managed care plan, and you need hospital care while you're traveling, you should call your insurer and ask about your coverage before entering a hospital. If you don't, your claim might be denied, costing you thousands of dollars.*

Before you go on a trip, check your insurance policy to see if you're covered while away from home and what requirements or exceptions there may be. If your coverage is through an employer-provided managed care plan and you'll be traveling to a city where the employer has another office, try to find out if any employees there belong to the same plan as you. If someone does, ask her to send you a copy of the plan's directory listing the health care facilities you can use. (This may sound like a ridiculous amount of trouble to go through, but I know of a California man who, while in Florida on a business trip, had a kidney stone problem and had to track down this information before he could enter a hospital.) Be sure to take your insurance card with you, too, so you'll have the insurer's phone number and your policy number handy.

If you're covered by Medicare

If you are on Medicare, your hospital care is covered by Part A, which most people age 65 and older get automatically. If you are age 65 or older and did not work enough quarters to qualify for Medicare, you can purchase Part A coverage for $309 a month ($170 per month if you have 30 to 40 quarters of Medicare-covered employment). For your first 60 days of inpatient care, you'll pay a deductible of $764. For longer hospital stays, you'll have to pay a daily co-insurance rate of $191 for days 61 through 90 and $382 per day thereafter.

Be aware that Medicare does not cover all hospital expenses. The expenses it won't cover include the following:

- The first three pints of whole blood or units of packed cells used in a calendar year in connection with covered services—unless the blood is replaced. (Your friends or family can donate the replacement for you.)
- A private hospital room, unless medically necessary, and a private-duty nurse.
- Personal convenience items, such as a telephone or TV in a hospital room.
- Nonemergency care in a hospital that does not participate in the Medicare program.
- Care received outside the United States and its territories, except under limited circumstances in Canada and Mexico.

If you are age 65 or older and you (or your spouse) are still working and covered by a group health plan through your employer, Medicare may pay only for Medicare-covered expenses that your employer plan won't fully pay. That is, your group health plan is your "primary payer" and Medicare is the "secondary payer."

Supplementing your Medicare benefits

Most Medicare beneficiaries buy supplemental insurance called Medigap, which is regulated by federal and state law. Medigap provides specific benefits that help fill the gaps in Medicare's coverage. You can find out what Medigap plans are available by contacting your state insurance department.

➤ **Recommendation:** *If you bought a Medigap policy prior to 1992, when Medigap plans became "standardized," your state might require you to switch to a newer plan. Check with your state insurance department to find out. Even if you're not required to convert an older policy, you should see if it would be to your advantage. Insurers must give you at least 30 days to review a*

Medigap policy and refund your premium if you decide you don't want the policy and return it within the "free look" period. Keep in mind, however, that, unless prohibited by your state, there may be a waiting period of up to six months before you become eligible for a benefit that was not included in your old policy.

Another supplemental health insurance product is called Medicare SELECT. It differs from standard Medigap insurance in that it requires you (except in an emergency) to use specific hospitals and, in some cases, specific doctors, to be eligible for full benefits. Because it restricts you to certain health care providers, this policy's premiums tend to be lower than other supplemental plans.

Note: Congress designed Medicare SELECT as an experimental program, which may be terminated in 1998. In that event, you will be able to keep the policy with no changes in benefits or, regardless of your health status, purchase another Medigap policy offered by the insurer. Also, although it's authorized for sale in every state, your state might not have approved it for sale. Check with your state insurance department.

If you don't have supplemental health insurance, you may be able to reduce your costs under Medicare by enrolling in a managed care plan. You can find out which plans serve your area by calling any Social Security office or your state insurance counseling office. The plan is required to have at least one 30-day open enrollment period each year during which Medicare beneficiaries can enroll without a health screening.

A few Medicare managed care plans offer a "point-of-service" (POS) option, which lets you receive certain services outside the plan's provider network. In exchange for this flexibility, expect to pay at least 20 percent of the bill. If you travel frequently, live in another state during part of the year or want to continue using a physician who is not affiliated with the plan, this may be a good choice for you.

More ways to save money

If you are covered by Medicare and your financial resources sink low enough for you to qualify for Medicaid, most of your health care costs will be covered. While you are covered by Medicaid, if you have a Medigap policy that was purchased after Nov. 4, 1991, you can suspend the premiums (and benefits) for up to two years. You do so by notifying the Medigap insurer within 90 days of becoming eligible for Medicaid.

Note: You do not have to suspend your Medigap policy when you become eligible for Medicaid. You should discuss your options with your state Medicaid office.

If you served in the armed forces, you and your dependents may be eligible to use VA hospital facilities or receive treatment at designated civilian facilities that is paid for, at least in part, by CHAMPUS (Civilian Health and Medical Program of the Uniformed Services). In mid-1998 CHAMPUS is scheduled to be replaced by Tricare, the military's new managed care system. The best source of information is the Web site for the Department of Defense's Office of Health Affairs: http://www.ha.osd.mil/tricare/tri2.html.

What if you do not have any health care coverage and can prove that you have a low income (but not low enough to qualify for Medicaid)? Some hospitals that have been given federal aid for construction purposes are required by law to treat needy patients under the Hill-Burton program. You can find out the names of such hospitals by calling the Hill-Burton Uncompensated Services Hotline (Department of Health and Human Services) at (800) 638-0742 or inside Maryland at (800) 492-0359. Similarly, hospitals that receive state aid may be required to provide "charity care" to indigent patients. Contact your state insurance department for details.

Last-ditch options

If none of the above options is available to you because you're not age 65, didn't serve in the military and haven't used up all your financial resources, there are still a few steps you can take to keep your costs somewhat manageable. These include:

❑ **Explain to your doctor** that you're paying your own medical expenses and are trying to keep costs down. Doctors tend to pay more attention to expenses when they know you're spending your own money.

❑ **Ask your doctor** which hospitals he uses, and then call those hospitals to see what they charge for room, meals and use of the operating room. Find out if the hospital offers a payment plan that lets you pay part of your bill on a monthly basis. Tell your doctor you want to use the hospital that offers the lower-cost cure and/or installment plan.

❑ **Don't enter a hospital** until the day your inpatient procedure is scheduled. That will save you the expense of an unnecessary overnight stay.

❑ **Find out if you can take** your own routine medication, such as aspirin, to the hospital. Some hospitals charge several dollars per pill for dispensing over-the-counter drugs.

Emergency admission

In an emergency, you don't have the luxury of choosing your hospital. This presents a different set of financial issues from those in a nonemergency situation.

Theoretically, a hospital must provide emergency treatment regardless of whether you're insured or have the ability to pay for your care. This merely means the hospital must stabilize your condition before discharging you or transferring you to another hospital. "Stabilizing" your condition does not necessarily require the doctors to perform any medical heroics. For example, if an ambulance brings you to an emergency room after a car accident, the hospital should at least staunch the bleeding before sending you to another facility for surgery.

Observation: *Watches, clothing, glasses and other personal possessions have a way of getting lost in hospital emergency rooms and during inter-hospital transfers. If you notice something is missing, ask the hospital staff to search for it or, if feasible, to contact the ambulance service. Odds are, however, that you've seen the last of that personal item and you'll need to file a claim with your property insurance company.*

As soon as possible, the hospital will attempt to find out what, if any, insurance coverage you have and contact the insurer (including Medicare and Medicaid) for authorization to treat you. If you are unconscious or otherwise unable to provide the necessary information, the hospital's policy

If Your Emergency Occurs Outside the U.S.

Several companies offer travel insurance that includes emergency cash, translation services, medical referrals and links to U.S. doctors. When abroad, you call a 24-hour hotline to reach a staff member, who will make doctors' appointments, hospital arrangements or, if necessary, air evacuation reservations to the nearest approved medical facility. Note, however, that these insurance plans often have restrictions on pre-existing conditions. Contact your travel agent for information about this type of coverage. Other sources of information include:

- Access America, (800) 284-8300
- Europ Assistance Worldwide Services/Travel Assistance International, (800) 821-2828
- International SOS Assistance, (800) 523-8930
- Medical Air Services Association, (800) 989-6272
- TravMed/Medex Assistance, (800) 732-5309
- USAssist, (800) 756-5900

may be to assign a social worker to your case until a family member is located or a guardian is appointed by the local court.

➤ **Recommendation:** *For a small annual fee ($10 to $35), organizations such as Medic Alert will keep your critical medical information, including physician and family contacts, in a regularly updated database. You also receive a Medic Alert emblem engraved with a member number that emergency personnel can call to obtain your medical data.*

Even if you don't have health insurance (or Medicare, Medicaid or CHAMPUS/ Tricare), your emergency may be covered by other insurance. For example, if you are injured in an auto accident, at least some of your expenses will be covered under your auto insurance policy. Similarly, medical emergencies arising from accidents may be covered under property or liability insurance policies.

If your medical expenses are the result of an accident, you should talk to a lawyer. Note that state and federal laws seek to encourage people to act as good Samaritans by exempting them from some measure of liability for any incidental harm they do. Thus, someone who comes to your assistance after you've been involved in a car accident may be protected under your state's laws from being held liable, for example, for breaking your arm while rescuing you from a burning car.

Generally, your insurer will control how long your emergency hospitalization lasts and what course of treatment you receive. Obviously, the insurer will try to make your hospitalization as brief as possible. In terms of your finances, this may be good because it limits your deductibles, co-insurance and payments for noncovered expenses. On the other hand, a too-rapid discharge could mean that you end up paying for home health care services or even suffer a relapse that sends you back to the hospital.

Observation: *If you disagree with your insurer about whether you are well enough to be discharged from the hospital, you have the right to appeal that decision. Ask your physician or hospital social worker to help you with the appeal.*

DON'T LET THE PAPERWORK KILL YOU

You may start receiving bills from the various service providers about three weeks after you're admitted to the hospital. If you don't have insurance, contact these providers and tell them you're paying your own expenses and would like to make arrangements for small monthly payments. Most providers will agree to this type of arrangement.

If you do have insurance, you may need to contact the providers who are sending you bills and give them your policy number and the insurer's address where they should send their bills. It's a good idea to send copies of their bills to your insurer, which will also notify the providers of the correct billing procedures.

➤ **Recommendation:** *Don't pay any bills until you receive written notification that your insurer is denying the claim. Under certain circumstances, such as the provider not following proper billing procedures, you may not be held responsible for paying the claim—even when your insurer refuses to pay.*

Caution: *Some providers tell patients that they need to pay upfront for certain medical services or equipment and say the patients will be reimbursed by their insurance carrier.* Check with your insurance company before you pay for anything. Often the providers don't know what benefits your insurance covers and are just trying to save themselves time and money. Unfortunately, it can take several months to get your money back if it turns out that the service or equipment is covered under your insurance policy.

Track Everything

Most insurance plans have a limit on the amount of deductibles and co-insurance that you must pay. Some insurers keep track of your payments for you, but it's a good idea to keep records of what you've paid. Here are a few tips:

- Keep blank insurance claim forms on hand.
- Make copies of everything you submit for payment and all correspondence with insurance companies.
- Keep notes of all phone conversations you have with your insurance company, including the name of the person you spoke with.
- Review your bills to make sure they're accurate.
- Submit claims for everything for which you are billed, including medications.
- Review what has been paid by your insurance company. This information may be sent to you on an Explanation of Benefits (EOB) form. Keep the EOB form with your copy of the claim and invoice.
- If your insurance company denies payment on a claim, find out why. If you believe a legitimate claim was refused, follow the insurer's appeals process.

If you have health care coverage under more than one type of insurance, the provider typically can bill only one insurer at a time. For example, if you're covered under a group health insurance plan and also have CHAMPUS/Tricare because you served in the armed forces, the hospital or other provider will first bill the group health plan (the primary payer) and then bill CHAMPUS/Tricare, your secondary payer, for any remaining expenses. While this is going on, you'll get copies of the bills being sent out. Wait until both your primary and secondary payers have paid their appropriate shares before you send any money.

Note: You may receive a letter from a medical claims collection agency saying you are required to pay an outstanding bill. You should check with your insurer(s) to find out if they received the bill and what action they are taking. It may be that the hospital or other provider did not know where to send the bill or that you have secondary coverage. Contact the collection agency and the provider and give them this information. That generally will stop the dunning notices from coming to you.

Activating your other benefits

Aside from your medical bills, you'll obviously need to pay your ordinary living expenses. Getting the money to pay for these will require you to deal with a whole other aspect of paperwork: your medical records, accident reports and any other documentation that shows what happened to you, the medical diagnosis, your prognosis, treatment plan and current medical status.

If you are employed, contact your employer or Employee Assistance Program rep to find out what forms you need to submit to take extended sick leave, if this available. If you have disability income insurance through your employer, find out what documentation is needed to activate your benefits. (If you have purchased disability insurance on your own, ask your insurance agent to help you obtain the claim forms or call the insurer directly.)

The best time to start collecting copies of your medical records is while you're in the hospital. Once you're discharged, you'll need to submit a written request for your medical records, along with payment for photocopying and mailing expenses, and may have to wait several weeks to receive them. If you continue to get treatment on an outpatient basis, make sure you get copies of your medical reports from every doctor and therapist you see.

When you submit your claim for disability income insurance, you may encounter what's known as **reverse underwriting**. This means the insurance company waits until you file a claim to decide whether there are any problems with your original insurance application that would entitle it to refuse your claim. It may take one or two months to complete the investigation, during which you may not receive any benefits. Once the claim is approved, however, you'll receive payment for all the benefits due you, dating from the first day you became eligible.

Making It Through the Long Haul

6

After about two months in the hospital, my husband was declared "functional" in all regards and sent home, even though he couldn't walk, bathe, dress or eat without assistance. Further, I was instructed not to leave him at home alone because he might fall and injure himself. During this stage of John's recovery, his long-term-care insurance paid home health care benefits, and it refunded part of that year's premium.

John's rehab continued on an outpatient basis until the insurer's 90-day limit was reached; at that point, the rehab program said John had "met all treatment plan goals." Upon his "graduation" from rehab, the disability income insurer stopped sending weekly benefit checks.

However, by getting his new primary care physician to write a referral for more speech and physical therapy, I was able to get the disability income restarted, which more than paid for the additional therapy not covered by the health insurance.

Rehab Benefits Often Fall Short

Concerns that victims of serious accidents and illnesses were being denied coverage for rehabilitative therapy that might help return them to the work force led many state legislatures to pass laws requiring insurers to pay for a minimum number of days of rehab. Typically, these range from a low of 30 days (as in Maryland) to a high of 90 days (as in Virginia). Rehabilitation includes therapy to improve speech, vision, gait, cognitive thinking and other basic skills, as well as occupational and vocational training.

Caution: *The rehab hospital treating my husband never explicitly stated that he was being released from the program because his benefits were exhausted.* Yet every patient in the program with him received a similar "graduation" certificate when their insurance limit was reached. Be aware of such euphemisms because they become a part of your medical record, which is a crucial source of documentation examined by your employer, disability income insurer, the Social Security Administration and others to decide if you are really disabled or merely a malingerer.

If you do not have health insurance—or your rehab benefits have been exhausted—you may be able to obtain low-cost rehabilitation through your state, county or city department of rehabilitative services. Unfortunately, these services, which are often provided under contract to the lowest bidder, have a reputation for being limited in scope and quality.

A large number of nonprofit and for-profit organizations have sprung up to meet the growing demand for high-quality, individualized rehabilitation and work-transition assistance. The for-profit organizations can be very expensive, charging as much as $500 or more per day for full-time rehabilitation in a residential facility. In contrast, the nonprofits generally offer free or low-cost rehab in your home or community, deriving their income from contributions and membership fees.

Are You Really 'Work Ready'?

Once you've exhausted your rehabilitation benefits, you're likely to feel under pressure to return to work. You may even have been told that you're "work ready," which often is just another euphemism for having no more coverage. The question, however, is: Are you really ready?

If you have sick leave on the books or are eligible for unpaid leave under the Family and Medical Leave Act and have not used up your FMLA leave during your hospitalization or convalescence, you should discuss a part-time schedule with your employer. You may have to get your doctor's certification stating that you need to rebuild your stamina before resuming your previous workload. (*See details on FMLA leave in Section 4.*)

Many employers offer flex time, job sharing and telecommuting options, while others may be willing to explore these avenues as a way to ease you back into the office. Large employers, such as the federal government and other public agencies, may also offer a leave-sharing program, through which employees can donate annual leave to ill or injured co-workers who have used up all their own paid leave.

Observation: *In order for my husband to participate in his employer's leave-sharing program, he first had to go on leave-without-pay. When he returned to active status nearly eight months after his stroke, he received close to 380 hours of donated leave, about half of which immediately went back to his employer as repayment for the sick leave he'd been advanced when he went into the hospital. The rest of the donated leave allowed him to work a shortened schedule, yet get paid for a full 40-hour week—until his health declined to the point where he couldn't continue working and had no more leave available.*

If You Can't Earn As Much As You Did . . .

In this case, you may need to supplement your income in order to pay your bills. Some of your options may depend on how much you now earn, while others essentially boil down to a systematic depletion of your financial resources. Here are a few suggestions:

❑ **Carefully review your disability income insurance policy** to see if it pays a reduced benefit when you have a partial or residual disability (*see Section 2*). If so, and your work situation fits the policy's guidelines, file a claim.

❑ **If you have a pension plan**, such as a 401(k), through your employer, you may be able to make a "hardship" withdrawal of your own contributions and, possibly, part of your employer's contribution. Check with your employer to see if there are any limitations on your ability to make future contributions and what tax consequences you may face as a result of taking out pretax contributions.

❑ **Rather than make a "hardship" withdrawal** from your 401(k), find out if you can borrow money from your account. You'll need to ask your employer about the length of the loan, interest payments and any other conditions that might be attached to the loan.

❑ **If you have opened a Roth IRA**, current guidelines state that after you've had the account for five years, you can withdraw up to a lifetime limit of $10,000 penalty free if you become disabled. However, it is unclear as of this writing how "disabled" will be defined in 2003, the first year when anyone will be eligible to make this type of a withdrawal.

WHAT IF YOU JUST CAN'T WORK—PERIOD?

Experts recommend that you at least try to work. You might be surprised by what you can do. But if it doesn't pan out, then you'll have useful documentation of your inability to sustain employment. This documentation can prove extremely valuable when you apply for government benefits. It may also entitle you to a new period of coverage under your disability income insurance.

Some employers offer a combination of short-term and long-term disability income insurance. After the short-term benefits are exhausted (usually after 26 weeks), you simply file a claim for benefits under the long-term disability policy. These benefits may continue for your lifetime, or stop when you become age 65 and begin collecting retirement benefits, or last five years or some other fixed period.

If you attempt to return to work while you are receiving disability income benefits through an insurance plan that pays only when you're considered totally disabled, you should expect your benefits to cease. That doesn't necessarily mean, though, that you can't get the benefits reactivated if you are unable to keep working.

➤ **Recommendation:** *In order to avoid risking a disability benefits cutoff, carefully review your policy to see (1) how long you must work before becoming eligible for benefits again, (2) whether benefits apply only to a "new" disability, (3) if there is a new waiting period after you stop working and (4) if there are any other restrictions that might prevent you from reactivating your benefits.*

Regardless of whether you have disability income insurance, you may be eligible to receive Social Security Disability Insurance (SSDI) income. Be prepared, however, for an exhausting application process, which is described in the next section.

Can Ill or Disabled Employees Be Forced to Retire?

The Americans With Disabilities Act protects covered employees from being fired just because they cannot perform duties that are incidental to their job (*see Section 4*). However, if your medical condition interferes with your essential job duties and there is no reasonable accommodation that can be made that would allow you to perform those duties, your employer is legally entitled to give you the pink slip.

If you are having difficulty getting your work done, don't let the situation get so bad that your employer's only choice is to fire you. Think about what assistance you could use to accomplish your work, or look into other jobs you could do for your employer. Or, request that your local department of rehabilitative services talk with your employer about ways to help you keep your job.

Sad to say, most people cannot afford to take early retirement. However, if your employer offers a "medical disability retirement," which may pay as much as 50 percent or more of your current salary (or average salary for the "top three" years of employment), it may be worthwhile to take the offer.

Caution: *Be aware that some medical disability retirement options require you to apply for Social Security Disability Insurance benefits and will deduct a percentage of those benefits from the retirement annuity.*

SOCIAL SECURITY DISABILITY INSURANCE

As mentioned in Section 2, the Social Security Administration reportedly turns down about 70 percent of the initial SSDI applications submitted. Many people blame the high rejection rate on Congress, which has defined "disability" for purposes of SSDI as:

> *The inability to engage in any substantial gainful activity by reason of any medically determinable physical or mental impairment which can be expected to result in death or which has lasted or can be expected to last for a continuous period of not less than 12 months. A person must not only be unable to do his or her previous work but cannot, considering age, education, and work experience, engage in any other kind of substantial gainful work which exists in the national economy. It is immaterial whether such work exists in the immediate area, or whether a specific job vacancy exists, or whether the worker would be hired if he or she applied for work. The worker's impairment or impairments must be the primary reason for his or her inability to engage in substantial gainful activity, although age, education, and work experience are also taken into consideration in determining the worker's ability to do work other than previous work.*

Social Security uses a five-step process to determine whether the above definition applies to an individual case. Basically, here's how that process works:

1. Are you working? If you are and your earnings average $500 or more per month, generally you cannot be considered disabled.

2. Is your condition severe? Your impairments must interfere with basic work-related activities in order for your claim to be considered.

3. Is your condition found on the list of disabling impairments? Social Security maintains a list ("The Blue Book") of impairments considered so severe that they automatically mean you are disabled. If your condition is not on the list, Social Security must decide if its severity is equal to an impairment on the list.

4. Can you do the work you did previously? If your condition is severe but not of the same severity as an impairment on the list, Social Security determines whether it interferes with your ability to do any kind of work you've done in the past 15 years. If it does not, your claim is denied. If it does, further consideration is given.

5. Can you do any other type of work? If you cannot do the type of work you did in the past 15 years, Social Security determines if you can do any other type of work, giving consideration to your age, education, past work experience and transferable skills. If you cannot do any other type of work, your claim is approved. Otherwise, your claim is denied.

Aside from this five-step process, your eligibility for SSDI depends on whether you have worked long enough to qualify for benefits. Generally, you must have worked five years to qualify. (The requirements are a little different if you're age 31 or younger because you may not have had sufficient opportunity to work.)

How much your SSDI monthly benefit will be depends on your reported earnings. You can request an "Earnings and Benefit Estimate Statement" from Social Security, which will indicate roughly how much your disability and retirement benefits will be.

Caution: *If you have earnings that you've not reported on your federal income tax return, your Social Security benefits may be significantly lower than they would otherwise have been.* For example, one person did not report her self-employment income and consequently is receiving monthly SSDI benefits of about $525. If she had been properly reporting and paying taxes on her income, her SSDI benefits would have been at least $1,215 a month.

How to Apply for SSDI

Not surprisingly, if you're disabled enough to qualify for SSDI, you're probably not able to get through the application process on your own. For this reason, many, if not most, applicants have a lawyer or claims counselor handle the procedure for them.

Indeed, Social Security expects applicants to be represented by attorneys and will automatically set aside up to 25 percent of your awarded benefits (or as much as $4,000) to pay the lawyer's fee. If you file your claim yourself, you need to tell Social Security that you are not using a lawyer.

Note: The National Organization of Social Security Claimants' Representatives offers a referral service: phone (800) 431-2804. In most cases, you'll be asked to pay only incidental costs, such as postage and phone calls, if your claim is rejected.

Although most people do engage a professional to represent them, it is possible to apply and have your claim approved on your own. (A majority of claims that were initially refused end up being approved on appeal. So if at first you don't succeed, don't give up.)

There is no waiting period for filing your SSDI application; technically, you could apply the same day you become disabled. However, there is a waiting period of five months after the month in which you became disabled before Social Security starts paying you benefits. In addition to the waiting period, it can take almost another two months before you receive your first payment. That's because you don't receive the current month's benefit until the following month. So even if you apply the same day you become disabled, you'd better have enough emergency funds to see you through the minimum seven-month period until the first SSDI check arrives.

Caution: *Because your disability must be expected to last at least one year, Social Security representatives discourage early filing unless there's obviously no chance of recovery.*

Diary of a 22-page application . . .

While writing this book, I handled my husband's claim, and it was approved in less than 60 days. Here's how I did it:

❑ **I researched the process** and learned that Social Security typically denies stroke victims' applications unless the stroke occurred more than 12 months previously or the applicant is elderly. The rationale is that, even though strokes are on Social Security's list of impairments, approximately half of all stroke survivors recover quite well, particularly if they are younger than age 50. So I decided to wait and see how my husband's recovery progressed.

❑ **So as not to cause my husband to lose any benefits** to which he might be entitled, I figured out what his waiting period was and, 11 months later, contacted Social Security. Thus I called in October 1997, 16 months after his stroke. In fact, I could have waited a total of 17 months but was afraid to cut the timing too close. Besides, at this point it was clear that John wouldn't be able to go back to work.

❑ **I called the Social Security Administration** at (800) 772-1213 and said I wanted to file an SSDI claim for my husband. I was given an appointment date at the local Social Security office and received a letter telling me what documentation to bring along. The letter itself was extremely important because it indicated the date I had contacted them. Social Security can pay you benefits for as many as 12 months prior to the date you first made contact, provided that you submit the actual application within six months of the date of the letter. This is called your "protective filing date."

❑ **Prior to the appointment**, I went to my husband's safe deposit box at the bank and took out the following: his birth certificate, our marriage license, the divorce decree from his previous marriage and the DD-214 forms showing the years he served in the military. In addition, I made copies of our income tax return for the year in which he had his stroke, his earnings statement for the four weeks or so he had tried to work in early 1997 and all his medical records since he'd been hospitalized (which filled five boxes). I also took a deposit slip for his checking account, which is where we had decided his SSDI benefits should go. The letter also specified that I needed my husband's ex-wife's Social Security number. Further, I'd been told to bring proof of the medications my husband was taking—I got this information from the pharmacy.

Observation: *Having collected the medical records ahead of time shortened the claim-consideration period by at least 30 days. However, the process of photocopying and sorting all the papers took about 25 hours.*

❑ **Also prior to the appointment**, I obtained a letter from my husband's employer saying that John had tried to work but hadn't been able to perform the essential functions of his job. This was at my own initiative, and I'm sure it helped in the consideration process.

Caution: *The letter I received from Social Security regarding my appointment date did not contain the actual claim application.* It wasn't until I showed up for the appointment that I learned they should have supplied me the 22-page application, which I could have completed and submitted then and there. Consequently, I was given the application package during the interview and allowed 10 days to complete it and bring it back.

❑ **I did not bring my husband to the appointment with me.** He wasn't required to attend, and I thought it would be best for him not to hear any of the negative comments I'd have to make about his post-stroke impairments.

❑ **After the appointment**, I spent the better part of a week filling out the application. It required information about employment, hospitalization, treatment plans, doctors' names and addresses, medication, etc.; explanations about how his stroke affected his ability to work; and basic personal data. It's important to note that I obtained a copy of Social Security's "Blue Book" description pertaining to stroke and used the key terms in my description of John's impairment. I also used the job description supplied by John's employer to detail what John couldn't do anymore.

❑ **The following month, my husband was notified** that a medical examination had been scheduled to assess his condition. Earlier, we obtained a letter from his own physician detailing his current medical status. We took the letter with us to the medical exam—which turned out to be a good move because the physician had not been provided the medical records I'd given to Social Security.

❑ **A few weeks later, we were notified** that my husband's application had been approved. In addition to receiving benefits dating back to when he first became eligible to receive SSDI, John will automatically get Medicare coverage after 24 months of SSDI eligibility.

Caution: *During the appointment with Social Security, the representative told me I would be named John's "representative payee."* I did not realize that, as a consequence, we'd have to set up a new bank account, naming him the owner but making me the only one who can actually access the funds. Further, I am now required to keep records of how the money is spent each month and submit my accounting to Social Security once a year. Social Security appoints "representative payees" when the beneficiary is a minor or is considered mentally incompetent to handle financial responsibilities. In order for my husband to get control over his own SSDI benefits, he would have to go to the Social Security office and request the appropriate form for his doctor to certify that he no longer needs a representative payee. In that event, Social Security would also have the right to review his case and determine that he no longer qualified for SSDI benefits.

Recognize that SSDI payments are not guaranteed to continue indefinitely. But they won't be yanked just because you try to go back to work. In fact, you can continue receiving SSDI payments while setting up a home business, going to school or pursuing other routes toward financial independence. Social Security does, however, have a schedule for reviewing each type of impairment, depending on the probability of improvement. In my husband's case, Social Security will review his condition approximately every three years to see if he's still eligible for SSDI.

WHEN YOUR CONDITION KEEPS YOU AT HOME

If you're essentially homebound by your medical condition, your long-term-care policy may pay daily benefits for hiring a home health care worker, homemaker or aide to assist you. Even better, some policies pay benefits when friends or relatives provide the assistance.

Without long-term-care insurance, your home health care can become quite expensive, costing between $8,000 and $20,000 a year, depending on where you live, for four hours a day, five days a week. You may also be responsible for paying the worker's payroll taxes, including Social Security, which can add more than $1,000 to the bill.

Because Medicare rarely pays for home health care, most people end up relying on friends or relatives. Another option is to trade room and board for live-in help; people living near college campuses sometimes find students willing to help around the house in exchange for a free room and kitchen privileges.

If you meet various requirements (age, income and so forth), you may also be able to obtain free or low-cost services through your area agency on aging, social services or local religious groups and volunteer organizations. These services include:

Helpful Tips

Your medical condition may qualify you for a surprising number of extra conveniences, including:

❑ **Absentee Voting:** Contact your local elections office for information about applying for an absentee ballot. You don't need a doctor's certification to apply. Moreover, if a family member is providing your home care, that person also can apply to vote by mail.

❑ **Disabled Parking Decal:** Contact your local Department of Motor Vehicles for an application. (Some hospitals also keep these applications on hand.) You'll need a health care provider's certification that your medical condition affects your mobility. You may qualify for either a temporary or permanent hanging tag or, possibly, a handicapped license plate. Some localities allow vehicles with disabled parking decals to park free in metered parking spaces.

❑ **Discount Fare Cards:** Contact your local public transportation authority for an application. You may need a health care provider's certification that your medical condition affects your mobility. You may need to have your photo taken for an ID card that will entitle you to reduced bus and subway fares.

❑ **Tax Assistance:** The IRS offers special assistance for persons with disabilities, including help with completing your tax return through the Volunteer Income Tax Assistance Program. Information is available in Publication 910, *Guide to Free Tax Services*, and Publication 907, *Information for Persons with Disabilities*. To order these free publications, call (800) 829-3676.

Adult Day Care: therapeutic, rehabilitative and support activities provided in a senior center or community center for a portion of the day.

Handyman Services: heavy-duty housecleaning, minor home repairs, yardwork, installing safety devices and winterizing homes.

Companionship Services: companion visits to isolated and homebound individuals; general light errands.

Escort Services: accompaniment and personal assistance for the elderly.

Home Delivered Meals: delivery of hot lunch and sometimes evening meals.

Home Health Aides: assistance with eating, dressing, bathing, administering medications, etc., as well as light household chores.

Home Health Care: nursing, social work, occupational therapy, physical therapy and other rehabilitation services.

Homemaker Services: shopping, laundry, light cleaning, dressing, meal preparation and escort services on medical visits.

Nutritional Programs: congregate lunch programs, which may also include recreational and educational activities.

Respite Care: temporary care provided in the home, at an adult day care center or other facility, to give relief to primary caregivers.

Social Day Care: supportive but not rehabilitative services (recreation, social work services, meals, transportation and, occasionally, health services) provided in an adult day care center or other facility.

Telephone Reassurance: phone calls providing contact and socialization for the homebound.

Transportation: travel by car or specialized vans to and from medical care, supermarkets, shopping malls, cultural events and so forth.

Note: Victims of brain injuries, including strokes, may have their driver's license revoked if their physician is required to notify the state Department of Motor Vehicles of the impairment. To regain your license, you would be required to take a road test. You may find it helpful to contact your local hospital to see if it provides preclinical testing, which may include a simulated driving pro-

How to Save on Medications

When you have a serious medical condition, it's not unusual to spend $300 to $400 a month on prescription drugs, vitamins and other pharmacy items. Here are a few cost-cutting suggestions:

Follow the instructions: Skipping or cutting down on dosages may save money in the short term, but probably not in the long term. For example, high blood pressure that's not kept under control can lead to much worse conditions, including heart attack and stroke.

Ask for generics: Ask your doctor to prescribe a generic, rather than a brand-name drug, if possible.

Compare prices: You'd be surprised by the differences in prices among pharmacies.

Try mail order: Find out if you can purchase your medicine less expensively through a mail-order service, such as that provided by the American Association of Retired Persons.

Join a "club": Some pharmacies offer discounts for "frequent buyers." For example, one pharmacy gives customers 10 percent off every Tuesday on vitamin, mineral and herbal supplements.

Get prescriptions filled at the same location: A number of pharmacies keep computerized records of all the prescription medications you buy. The computer may be programmed to alert the pharmacist to any potential conflicts when you get a new medication. This can save you big-time money by helping you avoid serious medical complications.

gram that tests your reflexes and cognitive ability. Commercial driver education programs also may be of assistance.

IF YOU'RE FACING A LIFETIME-CARE SITUATION

When the prognosis is that your condition will worsen over time, you need to consider your long-term options for health care. Costs for long-term care are growing yearly. In Section 2 we provided information about various options for paying the expenses. This section offers additional information about several possible long-term-care choices.

Continuing-care retirement communities

A relatively new option for long-term care, about 1,400 such planned communities are expected to be established by the year 2000. These can be costly to buy into, with prices from $250,000 to about $650,000, although there are some less expensive ones. Rental communities also are available.

Some continuing-care communities provide full nursing home care—some for only a relatively short period; others for a lifetime. Obviously, the more care that's included, the more expensive the entrance fee. Nonetheless, it can be worth the price because these communities offer peace of mind. Most aspects of living—from meals to long-term care—can be covered in the same contract.

There are three general types of contracts for continuing-care communities:

❑ **"A" or extensive continuing-care contracts:** These are the most costly and all-encompassing, providing unlimited nursing home care. The national median cost was $59,000 in 1993, but prices can range all the way up to hundreds of thousands of dollars. The price differences depend on location and amenities, as well as whether any of the entrance fees are refundable to your estate. In 1997 monthly fees averaged $1,500, with the range from $750 to $4,000.

❑ **"B" or modified contracts:** These provide less long-term-care coverage, perhaps 60 to 75 days per year with no additional charge. Residents would then be required to pay $50 to $150 or more extra per day. The national median entrance fee is about $42,000, and monthly fees run about $700 and up.

❑ **"C" or fee-for-service contracts:** These communities have access to long-term health care facilities, but you must pay the full daily rate. You're also charged for meals, housekeeping and other services. The national median entrance fee is $35,000, and monthly fees are about $600.

More than 90 percent of these communities are regulated under state law. In addition, some are accredited by the Continuing Care Accreditation Commission, located at 901 E St. NW, Suite 500, Washington, DC 20004; phone (202) 783-7286.

Assisted care/assisted living facilities

If your medical problems are not serious enough for you to enter a nursing home, you may be able to save about 35 percent of the cost of a nursing home by living in an assisted care or assisted living facility. The expense is still high—the national average five years ago was $1,765 monthly.

To find out about facilities in your community, call the Eldercare Locator Service at (800) 677-1116. You can obtain a list of accredited facilities from the Continuing Care Accreditation Commission.

A less expensive alternative is known as a board-and-care facility, which may house anywhere from six to 150 residents. The emphasis is on a homelike environment that tends to emotional, intellectual and social needs. Three meals a day are served in a common dining room. Nursing or other medical care is not provided.

TIPS ON SELECTING A NURSING HOME

The Illinois Council for Long-Term Care suggests that you ask the following questions when considering a nursing home:

- Is the home licensed? Ask to see the license.
- Does the administrator have a current state license? Ask to see it.
- Is the nursing home approved by Medicare and Medicaid?
- What other insurance plans are accepted?
- Are there provisions for 24-hour medical care?
- Can a resident use his own physician?
- Are there facilities on site for physical and occupational therapy?
- What is the level of training and staffing of the nursing staff?
- When was the last state or local inspection? What were the results?
- Are routine and emergency drugs available?
- Does therapy cost extra? If so, how much?
- How are residents' medical needs met? Does the nursing home have an arrangement with a nearby hospital to handle emergencies?
- Are call bells responded to promptly?
- Do residents who do not receive physical therapy have the opportunity for daily exercise and for walking with assistance?
- Are ombudsmen phone numbers prominently displayed?
- Are there handrails in hallways and grab bars in bathrooms?
- Are there access ramps for wheelchairs and walkers throughout the facility?
- Are there additional charges for personal laundry?
- Can a husband and wife share a room?
- Where is the residents' money kept? Are there provisions for personal banking services?
- What types of recreational activities are available? Ask to see the schedule.

THE BIG 'IF'

When your medical condition is terminal, usually defined as having less than six months to live, you may want to consider hospice care. Some hospices are based in hospitals, but many are independent and focus on enabling you to live at home as long as possible.

Hospice care emphasizes pain management but also addresses nutritional, physical therapy and spiritual needs. About 85 percent of those served by hospices have cancer, and the average length of stay in the program is nearly 60 days, according to the National

Hospice Organization. Medicare, Medicaid and long-term-care insurance generally pay for hospice care. Some health insurance policies may also cover it.

If you haven't written a will, you should do so before the state writes one for you. You may also benefit from talking to an attorney about setting up a living trust. This type of trust essentially removes all your property from your estate, avoiding the need for probate. You and your spouse may also want to consider setting up a bypass trust to minimize estate taxes.

Conclusion

Have you covered all the bases?

Every 15 seconds, someone in the United States suffers a brain injury, and one in 20 will become permanently disabled. If that person were you, would you and your family be prepared to cope?

Make sure you've done all you can to prepare for a medical catastrophe. At this point you may want to refer back to the checklist at the beginning of Part II. Make an appointment with your attorney to ensure that your will is up to date and your other legal and financial interests are adequately protected.

Whether you live alone or have a family, you'll benefit from all the help you can get. Make a pact with one or two friends to help each other out in a crisis.

Finally, keep in mind that caring for another person is a tremendous responsibility, particularly when it's in addition to a full-time job and other obligations. Consider the following statistics from the National Family Caregivers Association and other sources:

- *65 percent of caregivers don't receive consistent help from other family members.*
- *68 percent of caregivers are between the ages of 40 and 59.*
- *69 percent of caregivers say frustration is their most frequent emotion.*
- *77 percent of caregivers are employed outside the home at least part time.*
- *80 percent of caregivers are women.*
- *85 percent of marriages that are complicated by a chronic illness will eventually fail.*

***The bottom line:** Serious medical conditions affect everyone—not just the patient. There are many sources of information and assistance concerning various aspects of coping with illness, injury and disability. Don't hesitate to ask for help.*